Dr. David F. Fardon is an orthopedic surgeon at Knoxville Orthopedic Clinic in Tennessee. He is a past president of the Tennessee State Orthopedic Society and is the founder and director of the Knoxville Back Care Center. In addition to membership in many professional medical associations, Dr. Fardon has had several articles published in professional journals and has made numerous television and public appearances as "The Visiting Doctor" for a local television series sponsored by the Knoxville Academy of Medicine.

Free Yourself From Neck Pain and Headache

DAVID F. FARDON, M.D.

A SPECTRUM BOOK

Prentice-Hall, Inc., Englewood Cliffs, N.J. 07632

Library of Congress Cataloging in Publication Data

Fardon, David F.
   Free yourself from neck pain and headache.

  (A Spectrum Book.)
  Includes index.
  1. Neck pain—Treatment. 2. Headache—Treatment.
3. Exercise therapy. 4. Self-care, Health. I. Title.
[DNLM: 1. Neck—Popular works. 2. Pain—Therapy—
Popular works. 3. Headache—Popular works. 4. Pain—
Prevention and control—Popular works. WE 708 F221f]
RC936.F37 1983   617'.5306   83–11061
ISBN 0–13–330720–4
ISBN 0–13–330712–3 (pbk.)

This book is available at a special discount when ordered
in bulk quantities. Contact Prentice-Hall, Inc., General
Publishing Division, Special Sales, Englewood Cliffs, N.J. 07632.

Editorial/production supervision: Suse L. Cioffi
Cover design by Judith Leeds
Manufacturing buyer: Patrick Mahoney

© 1983 by David F. Fardon

A SPECTRUM BOOK

ISBN 0-13-330712-3 {PBK.}

ISBN 0-13-330720-4

10 9 8 7 6 5 4 3 2 1

Printed in the United States of America

PRENTICE-HALL INTERNATIONAL, INC., *London*
PRENTICE-HALL OF AUSTRALIA PTY. LIMITED, *Sydney*
PRENTICE-HALL OF CANADA INC., *Toronto*
PRENTICE-HALL OF INDIA PRIVATE LIMITED, *New Delhi*
PRENTICE-HALL OF JAPAN, INC., *Tokyo*
PRENTICE-HALL OF SOUTHEAST ASIA PTE. LTD., *Singapore*
WHITEHALL BOOKS LIMITED, *Wellington, New Zealand*
EDITORA PRENTICE-HALL DO BRASIL LTDA., *Rio de Janeiro*

This work is dedicated to my wife, Judy, whose sensitivity to human needs provided inspiration for the contents and whose sensitivity to my needs provided the atmosphere in which it could be written. It is also dedicated to all those whose efforts to make the world a better place give them neck pains and tension headaches.

CONTENTS

ACKNOWLEDGMENTS   ix

INTRODUCTION   xi

chapter one
FIRST AID   1

chapter two
POSTURE   15

chapter three
ERGONOMICS AND BODY MECHANICS   26

chapter four
DAILY HABITS   43

chapter five
PSYCHOLOGICAL FACTORS   47

chapter six
DRUGS AND ALCOHOL   60

chapter seven
WEIGHT AND DIET   70

chapter eight
SEX   79

chapter nine
RECREATION   85

chapter ten
OCCUPATIONAL AND LEGAL QUESTIONS   88

chapter eleven
EXERCISE INTRODUCTION   94

chapter twelve
EXERCISES FOR POSTURE   96

chapter thirteen
RELAXATION EXERCISES   100

chapter fourteen
EXERCISES FOR FLEXIBILITY   108

chapter fifteen
EXERCISES FOR STRENGTHENING   118

chapter sixteen
EXERCISES FOR GENERAL FITNESS   127

chapter seventeen
EXERCISE SUMMARY   137

chapter eighteen
ANATOMY   139

chapter nineteen
NECK-RELATED MEDICAL PROBLEMS   155

chapter twenty
BEYOND READING THIS BOOK   169

GLOSSARY   172

INDEX   187

ACKNOWLEDGMENTS

The unique feature of this book is the collection of many ideas into one volume focused on neck, head, and shoulder pain. Few of the ideas are original; they are derived from the accumulated experiences of countless medical and paramedical practitioners. They have been contributed, in the spirit of relief of human suffering, to the medical "literature" and oral tradition to which I make collective acknowledgment for most of the factual content of this book.

It has been my privilege to practice orthopedic surgery with a superb group of physicians at the Knoxville Orthopedic Clinic. Stimulus to give the best care for patients by innovative means has been provided by the energy of those physicians, the dedication of the employees of the clinic, and, most of all, by the patients who have entrusted us with their care. That stimulus has had a very direct influence on the writing of this book.

Faye Houston, who prepared the manuscript, did so with incredible speed and accuracy, under the most trying circumstances in that she simultaneously provided all the organization and public relations functions required of a medical secretary in a complex and busy practice. The dedication and good humor she sustained through it all were not only a service but also an inspiration.

INTRODUCTION

Five million doctor visits are made in the United States each year with neck pain as the primary complaint. Almost 10 million are made for headache, the commonest cause of which is related to neck muscle tension. Another 15 million are made for back pain, often related to neck disorders. Shoulder pain, again commonly associated with neck problems, leads to another 5 million visits.

These figures, taken from the *National Ambulatory Medical Care Survey*, don't count the millions who suffer without seeking help. Nor do they count visits to physical therapists, psychologists, chiropractors, biofeedback therapists, acupuncturists, hypnotists, health spas, school and work aid stations, nurses, or pharmacists. Nor do they count the efforts of lawyers, insurance adjustors, safety officers, social service workers, and vocational rehabilitation counselors who help deal with the occupational, legal, and social complications of neck injuries and head and neck pain.

Most of this is unnecessary. It is not in the best interest of society. It's not in your best interest, either, if you made one of those visits, traveling from one professional to another, seeking a cure that never came.

You may have had pains in the back of the neck; or tight throbbing headaches on both sides of your head; or a sore, painful area along the inner edge of the back of your shoulder blade; or

pains out along the muscles of the side of the neck and into the
shoulder; or any combination of these and other symptoms related
to neck disorders. Whatever was done for you may have made it
better for a while, but the problem kept coming back, and you
either gave up or sought more and different kinds of help.

Anyone with persisting neck and head pain needs help from
one professional. A physician needs to provide the reassurance
that the trouble is not coming from the heart, lungs, brain, or other
vital organ and that there is no destructive process such as a tumor
or infection present. That is likely to be the only help that is needed
from a physician or other professional.

Once reassured about the absence of a serious underlying
malady, you can and should take charge of the problem yourself.

A major reason so many people seek so many different kinds
of help is that they don't know what to do to help themselves. It
doesn't take medical or scientific knowledge. It just takes some
common sense, a willingness to work at it, and some easily understood information. This book provides that information.

One of the greatest difficulties with understanding neck and
head pain results from the search for one cause and one remedy.
This mistaken idea that there is just one thing wrong, and, that, if it
is fixed, the pain will disappear, is an easy one for the sufferer to
accept. The simplicity of the idea makes you want to believe it.
Unfortunately, it is rarely the case.

Practitioners of all types, because of the bias of their training
and experience, will with good intention encourage the acceptance
of this one cause–one remedy concept. The medical doctor writes
a prescription for inflammation, the surgeon removes an abnormal
disc, the chiropractor manipulates a crooked neck, the therapist
applies traction and ultrasound, the psychologist teaches control of
tension, and so on.

The practitioners' efforts often fail. Often, they judge that
they need to do more, so more and bigger treatments of the same
kind are tried. Finally, the specific area of discipline has provided
all it can and the patient moves on to another type of specialist—
perhaps off on another tangent of well-designed and well-meant
treatment that is doomed to failure—doomed because attention,
maybe too much attention, is given to a tunnel-visioned image of
the problem.

Claude Bernard, Nobel Prize–winning scientist, said, "the greatest error in the advancement of medical science has been the search for a single cause for a single disease." This is particularly true when considering neck pain and tension headache. It is an error made not only by medical scientists but by their patients, who explore their problem by looking through one tunnel after another without ever having a look at the whole picture.

By taking a look at the whole picture, the different factors that contribute to the problem can be identified. Many little remedies can be provided to address each problem.

In some cases, one or more of the problems may require a bigger remedy and may require the help of a professional. Usually, that is not the case. Even when it is, the chance of success will be much greater if the person with pain has a clear view of the whole problem and is making a full effort to provide self-care.

Accepting the responsibility for self-care is the best insurance against overtreatment or mistreatment by a professional. Those who understand their problem and are doing all they can for themselves seldom need professional help. When they do, the chances of success are much greater.

Accepting the responsibility for self-care is not just a matter of willingness. It requires confidence. Confidence comes from knowing how to look out for problems and what to do about them. That knowledge is what this book can provide.

The neck is critical to the functions of the back, shoulders, arms, and head. It is important to understand those relationships in order to understand how upper back and shoulder pain and certain types of headaches may be caused by neck disorders, and how pain in those areas can aggravate the neck condition.

The concept of "vicious circles" whereby a first pain causes a second pain, the second pain results in aggravation of the problem that caused the first, leading to the second's becoming worse yet, and so on, must be recognized. This circle concept can be applied to the many causes of neck pain, so that one can identify how posture stress, work stress, stiffness, weakness, tension, fear of pain, and the many other possible causative factors discussed in this book may all act together, revolving in circles that make each worse than it would have been alone—and leave you, the sufferer, in pain and feeling helpless.

Vicious circles are just the bad form of "positive feedback cycles." Healthful circles can occur, too. Flexibility, strength, proper body mechanics, good posture, and confidence in knowing how to control pain, relaxation, fitness, and many other positive factors are discussed in this book. A small gain in any one of these makes a gain in the others easier.

Sudden, dramatic changes as one hopes for in the one cause–one remedy scheme seldom occur. Recognition of the vicious circles and identification of their elements, along with establishment of healthful circles, change what has been getting slowly worse into what will get slowly better.

This book helps you recognize the problem elements. It gives you the knowledge of healing factors that you can set into motion for yourself. You may be wise to have those who are closest to you read the book, too, so they can help you with and understand your efforts.

This book does not provide a simple answer. If your problem is like that of most neck and head pain sufferers, you do not have a simple problem. This book provides tools to make things better. It also provides optimism. You can get better. It's up to you.

chapter one
FIRST AID

There are numerous treatments for neck pain. Many operations have been devised for surgical treatment of neck pain of certain causes. Many medicines have been used to relieve pain, relax muscles, reduce inflammation, and improve the general health. Direct injections of many different drugs, needles, and coagulation devices into many different sites of origin of neck pain are in use. The neck and upper back may be heated, cooled, stimulated by sound waves and electrical impulses, massaged, twisted, stretched, pulled upon, and manipulated in numerous ways. All sorts of things can be rubbed in, plastered upon, or bound around the neck. The mind's control over the body may be tapped by such treatments as psychotherapy, hypnosis, and biofeedback.

All of these treatments have worked for some people at some time. None of them work for everyone all of the time. All of them have a common factor. They require that some expert, some practitioner, do something to the person with neck pain.

This book will teach you the means of self-care of the neck. By correct application of the techniques described, neck pain should diminish. There may still be times, however, when neck pain flares and more than preventive measures are needed. During those times, first aid measures, self-applied, should usually solve the problem.

Confidence that you can handle your own neck care, even when problems arise, is an important part of solving the difficulties caused by neck pain. Fear of neck pain sometimes becomes a worse problem than the actual pain. You can learn to rid yourself of that fear by learning not only how to prevent the pain but to care for it when it occurs.

You will learn a great deal about the effect of different body positions on the neck. First, you should learn the positions that relieve neck pain, the "neck rest positions" (see Figure 1).

NECK REST POSITIONS

The neck rest positions are the positions that relieve the muscles of the neck from the work they are doing and allow the bones of the neck to assume the position least likely to put pressure on the discs and nerves. They can be assumed most effectively lying down. Since it is not always practical to lie down, a seated rest position is also described.

Supine Rest Position

Lie supine (on the back, face up) with a pillow under the knees. A more detailed discussion of neck pillows will be presented later. Use the neck pillow you find best suits you. If a pillow is not available, a small towel roll placed to support the curve of the neck and to be up under the base of the skull so as to tilt the head forward a little can be used (see Figure 1).

Pull your shoulder blades together in back and let the surface you are lying upon hold them there. Let the shoulders fall back comfortably and let the arms rest along your sides or cross them comfortably over your abdomen.

Seated Rest Position

When it is not possible or practical to use the supine rest position, the seated rest position may achieve almost the same effect. Another advantage of the seated position is that self massage (with

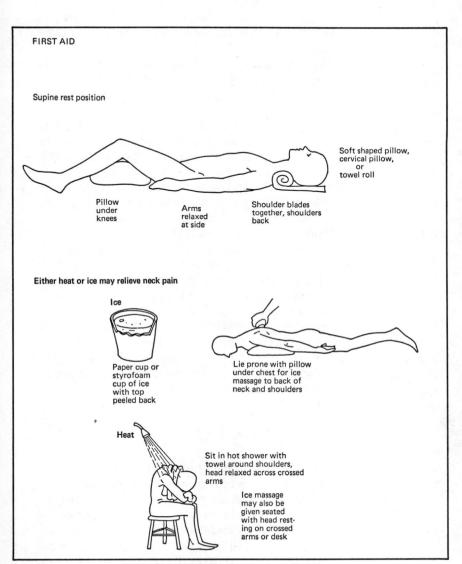

Figure 1 First Aid

or without analgesic balms or ice) can be accomplished at the same time (again, see Figure 1).

It is best to lean forward upon a desk or a chair back, especially if you are overweight through the abdomen. Otherwise you may bend forward at the hips using your knees to support your arms.

Sit in a comfortable chair with the knees at hip height or above and the feet flat on the floor. If your legs are short, or the chair too high, use a footstool or other support to bring the knees up while the feet remain flat.

Draw the abdomen in flat and draw the shoulders back, keeping the shoulder blades together. Bend forward at the hips and cross your arms in front of you. Let the crossed arms come to rest on your knees, or on the desk or chairback, if you choose to use one. Allow your forehead to come to rest on the middle of one forearm. Let the pressure against your elbows hold your shoulders back comfortably. Let your teeth separate and relax your jaw and tongue. Allow your eyebrows and cheeks to drop. Feel the muscles of the back of your neck relax.

You may proceed to do the relaxation exercises you will learn from either of these positions. You can free one hand to massage the neck muscles when in the seated position. Steady the forearm that supports your head by grasping the opposite knee or shoulder. Use the other hand to massage.

ICE MASSAGE

If you experience a sudden increase in neck pain with tightness or spasm of the muscles in the back of the neck and upper back, you may relieve it with an ice massage. Ice massage is especially helpful for relief of a sudden "crick" of the neck—pain and spasm of the neck muscles with a tendency to hold the head turned to one side.

Put a foam or paper cup full of water in the freezer of your refrigerator. When ready for use, pull off the top inch of the foam.

You may give yourself an ice massage in the seated rest position. It may be more effective to have someone else apply the ice massage to you, especially if the pain and muscle spasm are down near the shoulder blades. If you have someone else apply it, you may be either in the seated rest position or prone (lying face down) over pillows. Don't lie prone without sufficient pillows under the chest to allow you to bend the head straight forward and rest the forehead comfortably against the surface (see Figure 1).

Rub the ice gently around over the painful area for up to 10 minutes. As soon as you have finished the ice massage, do the flexibility exercises you will learn in the section on exercise. If your head has been turned toward one side and tilted toward the opposite shoulder, as in a "crick," try to sit or lie with it tilted and turned opposite to the way of the crick for 10 minutes or so, if the flexibility exercises have allowed you to do that without pain.

Ice may also be used effectively as an application, without massage. Put the ice in a plastic bag and then roll it in a towel and pin the towel closed over it. Drape the towel roll around the neck or across the shoulders so that it makes contact with the painful area. Leave it 15 or 20 minutes and then proceed with the flexibility exercises.

HEAT

Under most circumstances, heat and cold act as opposite forces. The effect of heat on tight, sore muscles is, however, very similar to that of ice.

The changes produced by ice may penetrate a little deeper and because the surface discomfort limits the time it can be tolerated, ice may be a little safer. Heat, properly applied, however, can be very soothing and can help with mobilization of tight muscles and joints.

Sitting in a shower in a rest position with hot water bathing the sore areas is a safe and effective means of heat application. Putting a towel over the sore area so that the shower water hits the towel maintains an even, comfortable heat (see Figure 1).

Heating pads, if used, should be used on low intensity. To avoid skin injury it is best to alternate 20 minutes of contact on with one hour off. The sensation of heat may be perpetuated by applying balms containing menthol, which are available without prescriptions from drug stores.

MANUAL MASSAGE, TRACTION, AND MOBILIZATION

Muscles of the neck may occasionally tighten and go into spasm suddenly for no apparent reason. This may produce a drawing to the side or turning of the chin toward one shoulder and up from it—acute "torticollis" or "wry neck," also sometimes called a "crick" in the neck. This may be present upon awakening after a seemingly normal day and night.

Tightness or spasm may also occur rapidly in response to fatigue, postural stress, or emotional tension. The muscles of the back of the neck may draw tight and seem to prevent normal position and movement of the head.

These situations may sometimes be helped by enlisting the aid of anyone who will help you. While heavy pulling and sudden jerking "manipulations" should be left to experts, if done at all, you can learn to massage, apply gentle traction, and assist with movement of a stiff neck. Having learned to do it, you can teach others to do it for you for first aid treatment of these cricks and tight muscles.

The person with the neck pain lies, supine, in the rest position except without any pillow. The massager stands or kneels above the head. With the fingertips of both hands, the massager gently pulls the muscles of the back of the neck from the shoulders up toward the base of the skull, lets go, and then pulls again. The fingertips stroke from the shoulders, up along the back of the neck, with the index fingers just behind the ears.

The person with the neck pain should relax more and more. The massager should very gradually pull harder along the back of the neck and base of the skull. Never force the head backward into extension (as though to look back toward the massager). This pulling with the hands along the natural long axis of the neck, as though to stretch the neck longer, is called "manual traction."

After a few minutes of this relaxing massage and manual traction, attempts at "mobilization" can be made. Mobilization is an effort to gain movement. Movement should never be sudden or vigorously forced.

The head can be gently moved into lateral flexion (so the ear

6

approaches the shoulder), into rotation (so the chin approaches the shoulder), and into flexion (so the chin approaches the chest). As explained elsewhere in this manual, some people should avoid extension (back of the head toward the shoulder blades), so this should be omitted except for those who know it is all right for them and should never be done forcefully for anyone.

Find the directions of motion that produce no pain. For example, if the chin is drawn toward the right shoulder, the head can usually be rotated further in that direction with no pain. Or if the ear is cocked toward one shoulder, the head can usually be tilted further toward that shoulder without pain. Repeat the painless motion over and over until the neck becomes more relaxed about movement, then gradually begin to try to move in the directions that caused pain at first. You want to stretch, perhaps causing a little discomfort, but never force to the point of causing pain.

Repeated, patient, gentle effort with massage, traction pull, and mobilization, first into the direction of no pain, will frequently loosen a tight, "cricked" neck and restore motion.

Once motion is regained in this way, it should be maintained by "active" movement; that is, the person with the neck pain moves the head by using the neck muscles. The movements that were regained with the assistance are repeated without help. If no one is available for help, you can sometimes do much of this on your own. The use of heat may substitute for a massage. Sit under a hot shower in the seated rest position, allowing the water to strike the sore or tight muscles of the back of the neck. Then rub some analgesic balm into the muscles and assume the supine rest position. Try to mobilize the neck by moving into the directions of free, painless motion at first.

If the neck pain is accompanied by pain down the arm or numbness in the arm, it may help to position the neck in such a way as to open up the nerve passages a little. Use the heat or ice massage first. Then lie on your side, painful side up. Put a small towel roll along the side of the neck, under the jaw on the nonpainful side. Allow the head to fall over the towel roll so that the ear on the nonpainful side approaches the shoulder. Turn the chin a little toward that shoulder. Stay in that position for about five minutes at first. Gradually work up to about fifteen minutes as tolerated.

If you suffer severe pain down the arm, especially of recent onset, do not position the head and chin toward the shoulder on the side of the pain. Always position them away. Also, don't allow anyone to try to "mobilize" your neck toward that side in such a situation.

Pain in the upper back from a sudden crick or catch may also often be worked out by massage and mobilization. Seated shower massage and heat are especially effective for pain in these "periscapular" (around the shoulder blades) areas. Sit straddling a chair and allow the hot water to run over the sore areas. Then twist the upper back while keeping the lower back straight on the chair. Roll one arm forward and the other back.

Move first in the direction of no pain. As motion increases, begin to move in the painful direction, slowly gaining motion. Leaning forward and backward and bringing the shoulders forward and backward as you rotate help vary the position to produce stretch in all directions. Avoid sudden jerking movements.

You may feel or hear a pop in your back or shoulders during the course of this that sometimes, though not always, is accompanied by relief of pain. It rarely is associated with increased pain. Usually it is just from the separation of joints that have been in tight contact, creating a little vacuum that causes the "pop." Frequently it cannot be reproduced right away. It is not necessary to hear or feel a "pop" for the mobilizations to help nor is a "pop" assurance that they have helped.

Massage of face and head muscles is particularly helpful to treatment of tension headache. The muscles are small and near the surface so the bulk of them can be easily massaged. They are also within easy reach, so self-massage is practical.

Massage is helpful in relieving the pain once it has occurred. It is also effective in preventing tension states. It should be part of the daily routine for those who suffer from headache, and, then, used in extra dose, for first aid.

Deep pressure over the muscles may directly stimulate muscle relaxation. Light stimulation of the skin over the muscles can produce reflexes that also help to relax these muscles. The sensation of face, head, and neck skin is very acute and the underlying muscles respond readily to skin stimulation.

The frontal (forehead) and temporal (side of the head) and the muscles of the back of the neck may be massaged using the finger tips. Begin over the forehead and apply deep pressure to the skin. Move the skin over the muscles, making small circles with the fingers. Slowly slide the fingers back over the temples, above the ears, and then down along the back of the ears, down the muscles of the back of the neck and into the neck and shoulder muscles. Think that you are pushing the tension and the pain out, that it is dispersing and dissolving away.

Use a brush with firm rigid bristles for skin massage. Plastic bristled shampooing brushes work well for this. Fingernails can be used if a brush is not available. Use the same motions along the same path as with finger massage.

MOTOR POINTS

The spots where branches of the nerves join the muscles are called motor points. These nerve endings may become sensitive when there is trouble anywhere along the nerve or too much stress and tension on the muscle. They are frequent locations of tender "trigger" spots.

Motor points conform, in most cases, to favored spots for acupuncture. A first aid form of this, called acupressure, can be applied and is usually done best by a helper.

Acupressure is done by pressing firmly, and continuously, on the chosen spot for three minutes. At first that seems to be a remarkably long time for both the patient and the helper, but it is important to persist for the full time. Relaxation and easing of the discomfort often occurs after a minute or two of frustrating absence of change.

The spots chosen for acupressure often, but not always, conform to the sites of the pain.

For relief of headache, points that are often successful sites for acupressure are located just above the top of the ear, directly in line with the ear canal; just in front of where the upper part of the ear attaches to the scalp in front; and over the bony knobs of the lower back of the skull.

Headache may often be relieved by acupressure over the motor points of the trapezius muscles, the large muscles that flare from the back of the neck down to the shoulder blades. Don't use acupressure on the front of the neck because of possible ill effects of pressure on the arteries.

Headache and neck pain may also sometimes be relieved by acupressure over the motor points out in the arm, a phenomenon that demonstrates the mystery of pain patterns and cycles related to head and neck pain. A favorite site for Oriental acupuncture, as well as acupressure, is the first dorsal interosseous, the small muscle that stands out in the back of the web space of the thumb when the thumb is squeezed tightly along the side of the palm and index finger. Another favored spot for neck pain is along the most distal crease of the palm near where the little finger joins the palm.

TRACTION

Traction means an effort to pull on the part, in this case the neck. Usually the major pulling effort is directed in the long axis of the neck—as though to pull it out so the head is farther from the shoulders.

As explained previously, traction can be applied manually, by a helper. This has limitations because help is not always available and the duration and force of pull needed often exceed the tolerance of the helper.

Traction devices are available for use at home or office. Doors, door casings, bed headboards, or hooks in the wall can be used to anchor the device. Pull is exerted through a strap around the back of the head and either the forehead or chin.

Traction stretches tense muscles and may break cycles of muscle spasm. It can separate openings in the bones, providing relief from pressure on entrapped nerves.

Traction does not help everyone and, in some cases, can make things worse. Those who have high blood pressure, heart disease, or history of stroke need to be especially cautious before using appliances that may put pressure around the neck.

Traction devices for the neck are not generally available to the public without prescription. This is for good reason—to protect the few people who might be harmed by them. If you have chronic neck and head pain and have no contraindication to the use of traction, your doctor will probably be willing to prescribe a home traction device for you if you explain your need for it. He may wish, and it may be wise for you, to try one out with the aid of a physical therapist to be sure you are using proper technique and to see if the effectiveness justifies the investment.

Many patients with neck problems need to avoid any forceful, head back (extension) positions. Special care to avoid such forces should be taken when using traction devices.

Pulling on the chin may cause pain in the teeth or angles of the jaw and may also be a sign that extension forces are being applied. If a chin strap is used, therefore, it must only be a positioner. You must be sure that the great majority of the pull is going through the strap around the back of the head.

Traction on the neck may be varied according to the device, the body position, the strength of the pull, the duration of the pull, and the frequency of the session.

Long-duration, "continuous" traction requires a device that can be attached to the bed, requires prolonged bed rest, and must be of low intensity. This is usually not practical for home care.

Short duration traction may be either "continuous" over a short period, usually 20 or 30 minutes, or "intermittent," meaning that the intensity builds up over a minute or two, diminishes to zero and then increases again.

Halters that wrap around the forehead avoid the problems of chin pull through the teeth and jaw. Some people have trouble getting halters to stay in place without a chin strap, however. Side straps should not squeeze the sides of the neck.

Hooking the traction device over a door provides a convenient, easily assembled means of fixation (see Figure 2). Most devices require that the door be open to allow hooking over the top of the door. A door stop or some stabilizing device needs to be used to keep the door steady. Face the door and place the chair far enough away so that the angle of pull is about 30 degrees. A chair with a good arm rest and back support is best.

For overhead "door" traction, starting with about 15 pounds

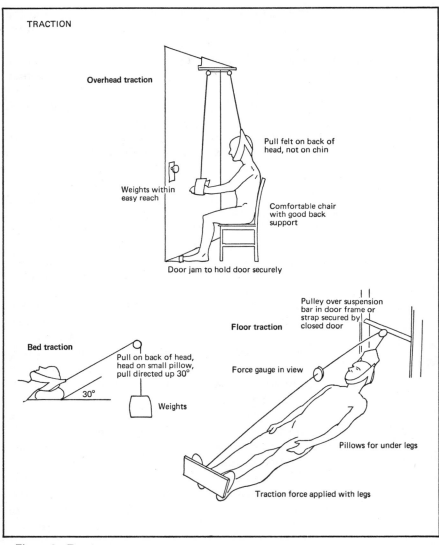

Figure 2 Traction

is best. This can be increased gradually over a few days to about 30 pounds. It is best to adjust the length of the rope and the height of the weight so it can be lifted on and off the lap.

A particularly safe and comfortable form of traction can be applied using the legs to control the force while lying down (supine) with pillows under the knees. The rope from the foot device to the pulley contains a gauge which can be placed for checking the weight. The disadvantage is that it is somewhat more complex to set up than overhead door traction. Angle of pull, force of pull, and duration of pull can all be varied according to your experience or doctor's prescription.

NECK SUPPORTS AND CONTACT DEVICES

Braces containing metal, plastic, or other rigid materials are used only for certain specific neck problems under a doctor's prescription. The soft collar, however, can be an effective first aid device, and is harmless when used properly.

Soft collars are made of felt or sponge rubber lined by an outer sleeve of cotton or synthetic material. Commercial collars fasten with a self-adhering fastener, but satisfactory ones can be made and fastened with tape or safety pins. If a commercial collar or suitable materials are not available, a rolled towel fastened with safety pins can serve temporarily.

The idea is to have some contact around the neck and provide some chin rest. The touch of any supportive device helps relieve muscle tension. The little bit of chin rest provided by a collar helps unload the neck muscles that control the posture of the head. The warmth provided may also have some positive effect.

In most situations, it is best to have the narrow side of the collar toward the front. This, of course, will vary depending on the width of the collar and the length of the neck.

The collar should not force the head back into extension unless the doctor specifically prescribes that it do so.

Collars provide comfort. They should not be relied upon to protect the neck from injury.

Collars are not very effective if worn for long periods of time.

They may interfere with proper muscle action and posture control if worn excessively. They may also be too dramatic a label of injury or illness resulting in undesirable changes in the way others treat you or that you feel about yourself. These potential undesirable effects of collars are not likely to occur when the collar is used occasionally as a first aid device.

The same effect of relief from tension by direct skin contact may be applied to headache pain. By relaxing neck muscles, a neck collar may indirectly relieve headache. Direct contact over the painful part of the head by an elastic headband, a hat, or eyeglasses may relieve head pain. For those who do not require vision correction, wearing plain or lightly tinted glasses with the temple pieces carefully fitted to provide comfort may be effective first aid for headaches.

MEDICINES

Excessive reliance on medication can be harmful in getting to the source of some of the important aspects of a neck and headache problem. There is no doubt, though, that some medicines can help with neck and head pain, particularly when the problem becomes acute.

Aspirin is one of the most effective pain and inflammation relieving medicines. It has the distinct advantage of being a nonprescription drug, thus falling in the category of self-care. Unless you have an ulcer, trouble with bleeding tendencies, or some other reason you cannot tolerate aspirin, the use of two or three aspirins four times a day for a few days may help. Your pharmacist can help you select coated aspirin to avoid stomach upsets. Combining aspirin with other nonprescription pain relievers seems to have no real advantage for most people.

Acetaminophen does not have the anti-inflammatory properties of aspirin. For those intolerant of aspirin, though, acetaminophen may give some of the pain-relieving benefits.

chapter two
POSTURE

Posture is the position, or attitude, in which the body is held. Neck posture determines the position of the head with its organs of hearing, sight, and smell, and muscles of speech and facial expression. The posture of the neck is, therefore, critical to the way people communicate with and perceive the world.

In order to maintain the head upright, the neck muscles must exert a constant pull. Even ordinary, relaxed activities require constant monitoring of the neck posture to position the eyes and ears for best function and to supplement facial expression.

When activity of the sense organs is more intense, the neck posture muscles are under even more tension. Driving, for example, requires prolonged maintenance of a certain neck and head attitude with constant readiness to make minor adjustments.

People who lead active, complicated lives feel the same tensions and need for alertness even when the situation does not wholly call for it. Such tensions frequently cause excess postural activity of the neck muscles.

The attitude of attention, interest, and alertness is one of the head being held forward, out in front of the shoulders. This posture along with the tension of readiness to make sudden adjustments puts a constant, excess stress on the muscles of the back of the neck and upper shoulders. These same muscles attach to the skull and may contribute to tension headaches.

15

Besides positioning the body for some current or anticipated action, posture serves as a kind of language to reflect feelings. Just as smiles and frowns are the language the mouth uses to reflect feelings, tense, flared neck muscles reflect feelings of anger or of fear.

Neck posture that keeps the head not only forward but bowed down a little is frequently combined with drooped shoulders and a stooped forward upper back. This is the posture of defeat, being overburdened, or fatigued—"having the weight of the world on the shoulders."

The result of such a stooped, defeated posture is increased strain on the muscles of the back of the neck and the muscles that support the shoulder blades (see Figure 3).

Another reason many people adopt a forward-stooped, neck-forward, shoulder-slumped posture is a holdover from psychological adjustments of adolescence. The years of rapid growth in adolescence are also years when many people don't want to stand out—they want to blend in and not be noticed. This may be a particular problem for people who grow very tall or for girls who develop large breasts. The attempts to conceal height or buxomness may lead to habitual posturing with head and shoulders forward and down and back stooped.

PINCH THE SCAPULAE

The most important factors in treating the problems that occur as the result of bad neck posture are an awareness of it and a resolution to control it. The solutions are fairly simple but hard to put into practice because they require breaking of old habits.

One key to proper posture of the head and neck is the position of the shoulder blades (scapulae). The scapulae move across the back of the chest to control the position of the arms in relation to the trunk. They can be felt to move across the chest by trying to draw the shoulders together in front of the chest and then "retracting" the shoulders back as far as they will go. As the shoulders are pulled back, the scapulae can be felt to come almost together in the

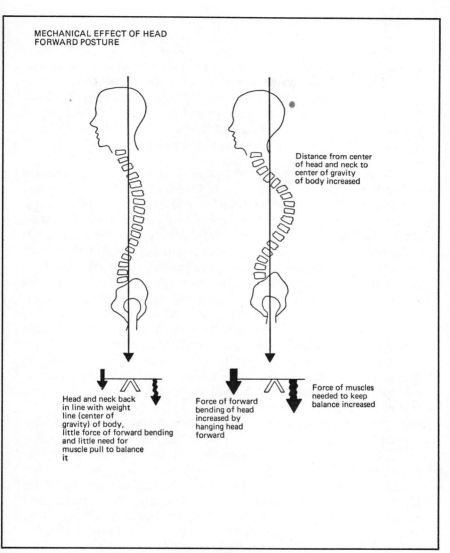

Figure 3 Mechanical Effect of Head Forward Posture

midline of the back, over the upper dorsal spine—"pinching the scapulae" together.

If you think only of pinching the scapulae together in back, the shoulders will follow and the neck posture will move to a position of less tension. If the shoulders are back, the neck will come back naturally and the neck muscles will not have to pull the head up as far to maintain a straight forward gaze. The lever arm upon which the 10-pound head is held is shortened and the work required of the muscles in keeping the head upright is, therefore, much diminished.

This scapulae-pinched, shoulders and head back position is the body language of confidence and leadership. That may be uncomfortable for people who have become in the habit of avoiding it. Once accustomed to it, however, many people enjoy the social rewards good posture can bring. Many people have maintained the body-language posture of adolescence from habit and no longer have the psychological needs for poor posture that they once had.

Full, easy movement and frequent changes of position are important aspects of posture. The reasons for emphasis on the scapulae-pinched, head and shoulders back posture are that it is mechanically advantageous and that most people with neck pain usually maintain the opposite posture. This emphasis is not meant to suggest that the head and shoulder back posture should be maintained constantly. Standing around like a military cadet for long periods of time is not a solution to this problem. Adopting that extreme posture momentarily and then relaxing about 20 percent from it helps to correct the bad posture and bring one toward the ideal.

Long-standing habits should not be changed abruptly. Awareness of the bad habits and knowledge of what good posture is and why it is important, however, can lead to repeated little adjustments, that eventually have a beneficial result. Changing bad habits is a matter of awareness and commitment to keep making adjustments in the right direction, never to slip back into old, harmful habits. The body and the mind take some time to adapt, so the continued effort to improve rather than sudden shifts works best.

GETTING TALL

The neck, being at the top of the spine, is affected not only by head and shoulder posture but by posture of the lower back as well. If the lower back sags excessively and the abdomen is allowed to protrude, the upper body has a tendency to lean backward. The lower neck compensates for this by bending forward, bringing the head back in front of the body's center of gravity. The eyes are kept straight ahead by cocking the upper neck backward. This all results in a strained posture of the neck. If the pelvis is tilted forward, the abdomen drawn in, and the lower back flattened, the correct posture of the neck becomes much easier.

A simple exercise to gain the feel of correct spinal posture is to "get taller." If you stand flat against the wall in a fully relaxed, slumped attitude, the curve of your lower back can be felt as the space between the wall and the lower back. The distance from the wall to the head and shoulders reflects the degree the shoulders slump and the excess flexion of the neck.

The correct posture comes from actually getting taller while standing in the same position. The abdomen is drawn in and the pelvis rolled forward as the low back flattens against the wall. The scapulae are pinched back so they can be held in the middle of the back by contact against the wall. The head is pulled back and the neck straightened to be as long as possible (see Figure 4).

An extension of this same exercise is an attempt to carry a book on the top of the head. This can be done with much greater facility if the head is pulled back and centered over the shoulders, the shoulders held back, and the spine held straight and tall.

The imagination can aid in maintaining the "getting tall" posture. Thinking of a wire attached to the top of the skull giving a gentle but firm upward pull gives a little psychological aid. Another aid is to keep a clear view for a "third eye," located where the knot of a necktie rests.

These little tricks and exercises for "getting tall" should be repeated throughout the day on a daily basis until the posture becomes habit.

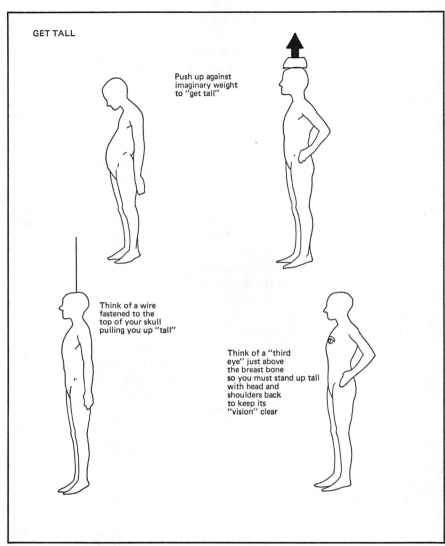

GET TALL

Push up against
imaginary weight
to "get tall"

Think of a wire
fastened to the
top of your skull
pulling you up "tall"

Think of a "third
eye" just above
the breast bone
so you must stand up tall
with head and
shoulders back
to keep its
"vision" clear

Figure 4   Get Tall

WHY CHANGE?

Changing posture habits is not easy even though most people can greatly improve their posture even with a single effort. Posture may be inherited or learned from an early age as evidenced by the remarkable similarity in posture often observed within families. The psychological aspects of posture and body language may take a long while to adjust. Physical adaptations have occurred that make it physically easier to do it the old way.

All of these things make keeping the old habits easier. They must be balanced by the desire to relieve or prevent the pain and other symptoms that are caused by the old posture habits. It is very tempting to seek the solution in some pill or manipulation or other formula that someone offers. No one else, however, can solve the problems that people create with their own bad posture habits.

One of the problems of changing posture is that it may require more muscular effort at first. Posture habits become lazy habits. We learn to lean on the ligaments and discs so we don't have to use our muscles. That is part of the reason that changing posture habits may seem "unnatural" and a lot of effort at first.

What is gained, of course, is freedom from the pain and the effects of progressive unhealthful changes in the spine. Healthy use of muscles is good for them. They can be conditioned to accept the extra work without causing discomfort. That is one reason strengthening exercises must be combined with posture training to achieve freedom from neck pain.

POSTURE IN LYING

To avoid sudden twisting stress to the neck and to avoid increased pain when the neck is already hurting, it is best to develop a habit of lying down in a certain way.

Sit on the side of the bed. Pinch the scapulae and draw the head back straight above the shoulders. Have the bed clear of pillows or other obstructions except for one small pillow at the head. Lean directly sideways making contact with the side of the shoulder and swing the bent knees and legs up onto the bed. From there either make minor comfort adjustments and stay in the side-lying position or roll to the back or other side.

Sleeping should be done on the side or on the back. Sleeping or lying for long in the prone (on the stomach) posture causes too much twisting stress to the neck. For short-term prone positioning, as for a massage, put enough pillows under the chest so that the forehead can rest on the bed and still allow for comfortable breathing without need to twist the neck.

The same kind of pillow is not right for everyone, but some generalities do apply to most everyone. Use of more than one pillow or use of a large, springy foam pillow puts too much forward push on the head without giving the curve of the neck enough support.

A small, loosely filled feather or synthetic particle filled pillow that will adapt easily to the shape of the head is satisfactory for most people. Some prefer no pillow at all, just using a small towel under the neck.

"Cervical pillows" of various types are commercially available. One type is a small cylinder shaped foam pillow that is to be put under the neck and allowed to bend around the side of the face and jaws without contacting the back of the head. Another type provides an inch or two of foam for under the head and three to four inches for under the neck. Either of these, as with a single, loosely filled feather pillow, can be adapted for neck support without excessive head pressure in either the supine (on the back) or lateral (on the side) sleeping posture.

It is important for people with neck pain to provide good postural care for the lower back as well as the neck. For on-the-back sleeping, a pillow under the knees may help prevent or relieve low back pain. Some people do better to put a small flat pillow or small towel roll in the curve of the lower back while sleeping supine.

There is no one right "orthopedic" mattress for people with neck and back pain. Individual preference with consideration to how it feels, durability, appearance, and affordability should be given rather than regarding the mattress as a medically prescribed item. Generally, the mattress should be firm but not rigid. The floor is too hard and a sagging mattress is too soft. A three-quarter-inch board cut to fit under the mattress may firm up an otherwise good one that has become too soft. A bed board may serve as a way to vary the hardness a little from time to time to find what works best. Good box springs and a reasonably firm mattress usually make bed boards unnecessary, however.

After lying down for a long time, particularly after sleeping the night, take a few minutes to loosen the neck up before arising. Turn the chin from one shoulder, across the chest as though wiping the chin on the chest, to the other shoulder. Touch the finger tips together in the back of the neck and pull gently against the muscles of the back of the neck and lean the head back, gently. Tilt the head to each side to touch the ear to the shoulder. Pinch the shoulder blades together and draw the shoulders back.

After loosening the neck, stretch the low back by pulling each knee up, drop the feet over the side and push to sitting position. All the while, hold the head and shoulders back.

Besides resting and sleeping, many people wish to lie down for reading or watching television. These practices can't really be recommended for people with neck pain, but, if they are to be done at all, they can be done in ways to reduce the chances of aggravating a neck problem.

Use of multiple pillows to prop yourself up for reading or watching television should be done in a way to avoid excessive pressure on the back of the head. The curve of the neck should be supported. A soft cervical collar may be helpful during such activity.

You can lie flat or nearly flat and watch television or read by using prism glasses. Lying on the side with the head properly supported may be satisfactory if the television is put near eye level.

STANDING POSTURE

The important features of good standing posture are keeping the head back over the shoulders, keeping the shoulders back with the scapulae pinched together, and keeping the abdomen in and the lower back flat. Being able to lift one foot up on something or being able to lift one arm on something at chest height helps maintain this posture comfortably.

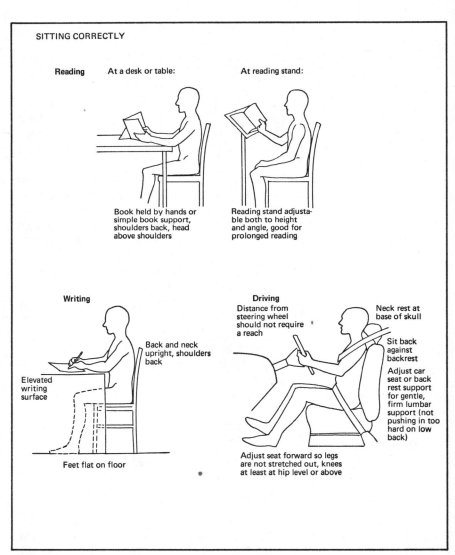

Figure 5 Sitting Correctly

24

SITTING POSTURE

Neck pain diminishes or can be prevented by sitting "tall," or upright with head and shoulders back and lower back supported. Arm rests on the chair or the use of a desk to support an arm at chest level helps to maintain this posture (see Figure 5).

Those who wear glasses should use reading glasses rather than bifocals. Straining the neck to keep the glasses in the correct position for the needed use is a common consequence of wearing bifocals.

More discussion of various aspects of standing and sitting posture follows in the next section on "ergonomics"—the ways of getting the body to perform work properly.

chapter three
ERGONOMICS AND BODY MECHANICS

Ergonomics is the science that studies the ways work is accomplished. Work in that sense and the sense we will use it means the spending of energy to create movement. The techniques of using the body to produce work we will call "body mechanics."

Work doesn't have to mean a job in the sense of what people get paid for. It certainly doesn't have to mean something unpleasant. It may include all the things you want to do as well as what you feel you should do.

STANDING WORK

The discussion of posture included proper techniques of standing. Work that requires standing should be done as much as possible following those techniques. It is important to try to avoid forward leaning with both feet flat on the floor.

Shaving or brushing teeth while leaning over a low sink are classic examples of poor body mechanics. Bathroom sinks and washbowls are too low to be used as a work surface. Mirrors behind the washbowl that require forward bending for close attention to shaving or makeup force the upper body to rotate out in front of the lower back, greatly increasing neck and lower back stress. An

26

extensible or hand mirror, for close observation, and avoiding the habit of unnecessarily close facial inspection save you from these stresses. Placing a stool under the washbowl or opening an under-the-sink cabinet door so one foot can be placed on a shelf allows you to get one foot up and the forward weight on it, placing the spine in a more balanced position.

So, you can see, body mechanics can become important from the first acts of the day (see Figure 6). Attention to the details of body mechanics with such things as early morning tooth brushing and shaving not only gets you off to a good start by not aggravating the neck early in the morning but establishes the habit of attending to the details of proper body mechanics. The same principles that apply to proper tooth brushing apply to many tasks performed standing throughout the day.

You may not want to redesign your bathroom sink because it is lower than the ideal work surface since you spend only a few minutes there each day. If you spend hours a day at the kitchen sink, cooking surface, work bench, or work table, though, the surface height is very important (see Figure 7). It should not be so low that you have to lean over nor so high that you cannot comfortably rest your elbows on it. Ideally either the work surface height or your standing surface can be varied a little from time to time. That changes the angle that your head must bend to observe the work material and the level of the hand and arm rests. Using a cutting board to raise the work surface or using a standing stool to raise your standing height may suffice if more adjustable equipment is not available. A high stool to allow periodic partial sitting may also help.

LIFTING AND BENDING

Many tasks require the transfer of materials from one surface height to another while standing. This may involve complex movements that require both lifting and twisting efforts. Proper lifting techniques must be learned first.

Lifting injuries are most often thought of as low back injuries. The entire spine works with lifting. Protection of the lower back by proper lifting techniques protects the neck as well.

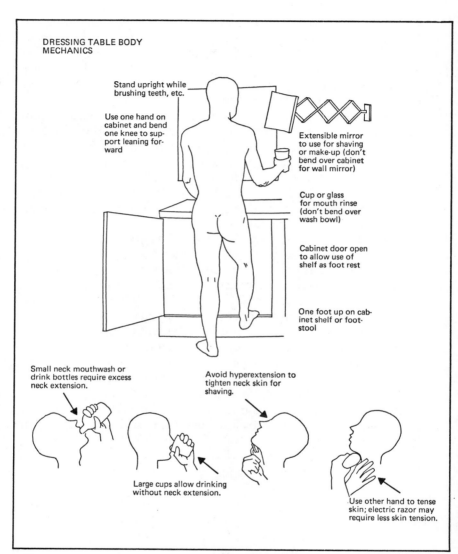

DRESSING TABLE BODY
MECHANICS

Stand upright while
brushing teeth, etc.

Use one hand on
cabinet and bend
one knee to sup-
port leaning for-
ward

Extensible mirror
to use for shaving
or make-up (don't
bend over cabinet
for wall mirror)

Cup or glass
for mouth rinse
(don't bend over
wash bowl)

Cabinet door open
to allow use of
shelf as foot rest

One foot up on cab-
inet shelf or foot-
stool

Small neck mouthwash or
drink bottles require excess
neck extension.

Avoid hyperextension to
tighten neck skin for
shaving.

Large cups allow drinking
without neck extension.

Use other hand to tense
skin; electric razor may
require less skin tension.

Figure 6   Dressing Table Body Mechanics

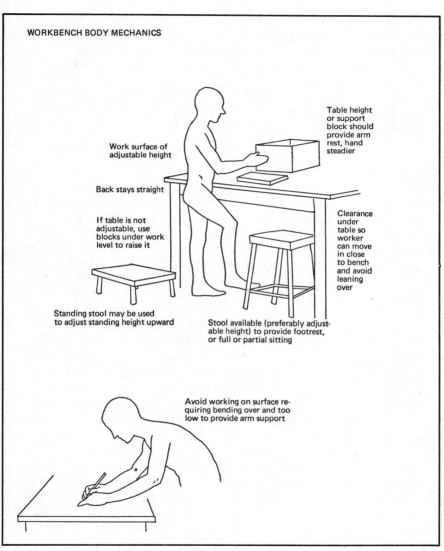

WORKBENCH BODY MECHANICS

Work surface of adjustable height

Table height or support block should provide arm rest, hand steadier

Back stays straight

If table is not adjustable, use blocks under work level to raise it

Clearance under table so worker can move in close to bench and avoid leaning over

Standing stool may be used to adjust standing height upward

Stool available (preferably adjustable height) to provide footrest, or full or partial sitting

Avoid working on surface requiring bending over and too low to provide arm support

Figure 7   Workbench Body Mechanics

29

The amount of weight that can be safely lifted depends on a large number of factors. There are, in fact, so many factors that to assign a limit in terms of pounds has very little meaning.

The size, shape, and texture of the objects are important variables. How far it must be lifted and from what height, whether it must be carried, and whether twisting and turning are involved in the lift all must be considered. The number of times the lift must be accomplished is another important factor.

HEAVY LIFTING

Lifting large, heavy objects from floor level is most efficiently accomplished by using the back for at least some of the lifting effort. If you squat down, bring the object in next to your body, lift it to chest level with your arms, and then rise to standing by lifting with your legs, you can lift rather heavy objects with very little stress to the lower back and to the neck. You should learn this lifting technique and use it for occasional heavy lifting. Most people, however, find this lifting technique too inefficient (and perhaps too hard on the knees) to use for repeated heavy lifting.

Repeated lifting of large, heavy objects is difficult, regardless of what techniques are mastered. To be able to accomplish such a task on a regular basis you need to be exceptionally fit. This kind of fitness goes beyond body mechanics and will be discussed elsewhere in this book. Here we want to emphasize mastery of the techniques to avoid injury from occasional heavy lifting or repeated lighter lifting.

Before the lift is attempted, make a careful evaluation of the task. Feel for the most secure hand-hold positions. Be sure the object is stable and won't suddenly shift after you have lifted it. Be sure the path to where you are going to place it is clear. Test the weight to make sure you can handle it before you commit yourself to the lift. If you can't handle it, get help. Even if you think you can handle it alone, if equipment or help is available, use them.

When squatting to pull an object in close, either at a full or partial squat, it is better to have one foot forward of the other. Using the hand opposite the forward foot as the leading hand balances the forces best. This creates a "diagonal" effect of the forces, minimizing twisting stress on the spine. This is a comfortable and effective way to deal with lifting and push-pull stresses, and, once learned, will be easy to make into a habit.

It is important to emphasize you should keep the weight of the object in close to your body. Experiments have been done in which instruments to measure the stress on discs and other structures in the lower back have been used on volunteers. These and other experiments repeatedly show that the greatest stresses are caused by efforts to lift objects held out away from the body. Bringing the object in close and moving the feet to minimize twisting do more than anything to decrease lifting stress on the spine.

Twisting during a lift shifts the stress to vulnerable areas. Whenever possible, it is best to gain full control of the weight, stand and turn, then set it down, rather than trying to rotate from one position to another by twisting. This, too, depends on fitness. Some activities, such as prolonged shoveling, can be accomplished efficiently only by twisting with heavy loads. Such activities can be done safely for long periods only by exceptionally fit people. Those less fit may learn to do such things by doing them less frequently, for shorter periods of time, and by compromising efficiency.

Don't lift what is clearly beyond what you are accustomed to doing. Except in rare emergencies, it is not worth the risk. Two people can lift much more safely than one. Repeated very heavy lifting should be done with equipment.

INTERMEDIATE LIFTING

Many people who have had back or neck trouble can regularly work at jobs or return to activities that require a moderate amount of lifting. To do so they must learn and practice proper techniques and be careful to keep themselves fit for the task.

The muscles of the buttocks, the hip extensors, can be quite strong. If they are exercised to keep strong they can bear much of the brunt of fairly heavy lifting. One of the reasons it is important to bend the hips and knees when lifting is that these muscles are positioned to be able to function with greatest strength when the hips are flexed. Bending hips and knees also serve as a means of getting the weight in closer to the body, thereby decreasing the leverage the weight has against the lower back. Control of the knee and power to lift the weight by straightening the knees depend on strong thigh muscles.

The muscles of the shoulders and arms must be able to handle the weight once a stable base is provided by proper positioning and use of the hip and leg muscles. Keeping the weight under control so balance is not lost is the job of strong arm and shoulder muscles. Adjustment of the height and position of the weight by strong arm muscles can keep the stress where it is best tolerated by the spine or can move it a little to shift the stress from spot to spot.

If the shoulder, arm, hip and leg muscles are conditioned for the task, a great deal of weight can be lifted and strenuous work accomplished without much stress to the spine. Much more can be accomplished safely if the proper techniques are learned, with special emphasis on keeping the load in close and avoiding excessive bending and twisting.

LIGHT LIFTING

When you bend over to lift a very light object, the problem is the bend rather than the weight of the lift. Put all of the weight well balanced on the forward leg. As you grasp the object, lift the rear leg clear off the floor, using it as a counter balance lever. If a hand hold is available, steady one hand at knee level and grasp the object with the other hand.

Setting Objects Down

In the process of lifting, holding, and setting down weights, it is always best to avoid the standing, feet flat and together position. Keep one foot forward. When standing still or preparing to walk with an object, have most of the weight on the back foot.

When setting an object down, it is best to try to get the forward foot as near the height of the surface as practical, to avoid leaning forward with the weight. An example is setting a grocery bag in an automobile trunk. Putting the forward foot, or even the knee, on the bumper may considerably unload the spine as the bag is lowered into the trunk. When possible, it is best to get the forward knee in under the surface, as when setting an object on a desk or table with a clear space under it.

The worst posture for the neck is adopted when the object is out in front of the body, the body is bent forward, and the neck is in an awkward, extended, head-up position. Such a posture might easily be adopted when leaning over to set a grocery bag into a car seat or trunk. Learn to take extra precautions to avoid stress in that posture.

Stooping and Bending

Bending or stooping down can be hard on the neck and on the lower back. The neck is put under particular stress if the head is extended, such as when you look into a low drawer while bending over. Squatting, kneeling or using a low chair or stool to sit upon while searching or reaching for low objects save on neck stress.

LIFTING ON THE JOB

Certain occupations are clearly safe as far as lifting restrictions are concerned and some are clearly hazardous. In between, many require decisions on the part of an employee and the employer on whether the particular job can be done effectively and safely by the particular employee. This is where body build, age, level of fitness, and knowledge of techniques all make a difference. The National Institute of Occupational Safety and Health provides guidelines on what is considered very safe and what is very hazardous. The zone in between, however, is left to the judgment of the employer and employee. You must make the decision as it applies to you, based on what is best for your health. You must make similar decisions about job activities not regulated by government agencies, such as housework, and nonoccupational stresses, such as yard work, gardening, and recreational sports.

PUSHING AND PULLING

Much of the focus on causes of neck and back pain is placed on lifting. Pushing and pulling may also produce back and neck stress. The essential features of safety are the same: keep control of the situation; do not try what is beyond what you are accustomed to doing; keep one foot in front of the other; use the "diagonal" stress principles to balance your body and the force you are exerting; bend the knees, and try to keep the hand near shoulder level. When you have a choice, pushing can be done with less back and neck stress than pulling. Get the forward leg or shoulder against the object to assist with the push. Avoid twisting movements where possible.

REACHING AND WORKING OVERHEAD

Reaching, lifting above chest level, and working with the hands above eye level cause particular problems for the neck. The head back, or "extended," posture of the neck is an awkward, uncomfortable one for most people and a dangerous one for some.

Reaching up to lift heavy objects down from a shelf creates several unique hazards. Preparation to avoid the injuries that may result could save a few moments of pain or a lifetime of disability (see Figure 8).

A stable ladder, stool, or platform should be secured and properly positioned so that the chest may be brought as close as possible to the height of the object. A clear stable way must be secured up and down the ladder and to the site where the object is to be set.

The object should be carefully inspected to determine its size, texture, hand holds, internal stability, integrity of its container, and weight before committing to the lift. Get help or equipment if there is a doubt that you can handle it.

Have the pelvis tilted and one leg in front of the other when making the lift. Keep the neck straight and the chin tucked in. Lift with the arms and bring the weight of the object against the chest, not the side of the head and neck.

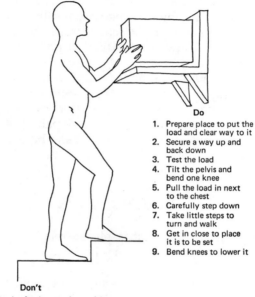

LIFTING DOWN FROM
A HEIGHT

Do

1. Prepare place to put the load and clear way to it
2. Secure a way up and back down
3. Test the load
4. Tilt the pelvis and bend one knee
5. Pull the load in next to the chest
6. Carefully step down
7. Take little steps to turn and walk
8. Get in close to place it is to be set
9. Bend knees to lower it

Don't

1. Take on loads of unknown size, weight, or distribution
2. Lift down from above head
3. Let back sway in as weight comes down
4. Let neck extend as weight is held
5. Twist to set the load down

Figure 8 Lifting Down from a Height

Carefully back down, keeping the back flat and the feet well-balanced. Be sure each new foot placement is secure before shifting the body weight to it.

Once down, take small steps to turn toward the destination. Avoid twisting.

Improper execution of such tasks is a common cause of sudden cricks and strains among otherwise healthy people. For those with arthritic or "spondylosis" changes in the cervical spine, a sudden blow or fall in a neck extended position could result in permanent paralysis.

Work that requires prolonged effort above chest level, such as painting a ceiling or trimming trees, should be done with special tools to extend the arm reach. Extra effort to provide ladders or scaffolds will be well worth it for the neck pain it saves. Those not accustomed to doing such tasks on a regular basis should perform them in short segments with frequent breaks for flexibility exercises.

SITTING WORK

The choice of where the seat is placed relative to what is to be viewed or worked upon determines how much stress will be on the neck.

If attention must be paid to action at or above eye level, but at a distance from where you are sitting, then it is best to make sure that distance is great enough to allow the head and neck to be in a comfortable, nearly neutral posture. Sitting up close to the screen in theatres or close to the blackboard in classrooms puts undue stress on the neck. Sitting further back, even if glasses are necessary to improve the perception of what is presented, allows more freedom of neck movement and a more comfortable, neutral posture.

The seat itself needs to be chosen to provide good spinal support through the lower back. Arm rests may help with tension on shoulder muscles. A footstool or chair rung to allow elevation of one foot may help the spinal posture.

In doing close-up work, such as writing at a desk or typing, being able to vary the height of the chair (see Figure 9), the desk,

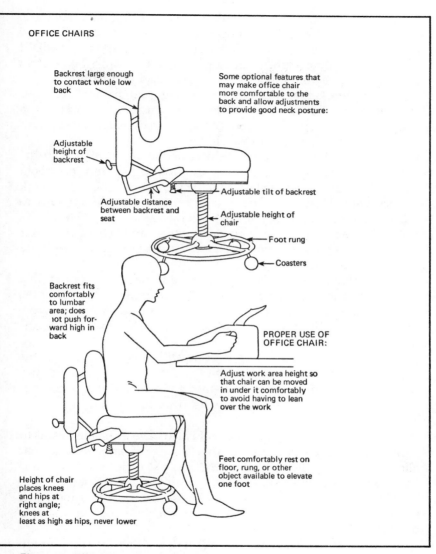

Figure 9 Office Chairs

the object that is being worked upon, or some combination of those factors may be helpful. Prolonged activity in the same forward leaning posture leads to muscle fatigue and tension with resultant neck and shoulder pain. Changing the level spreads the stresses around a little before one level is overstressed and painful.

If the work chair does not have height adjustment features, the height can be varied by using sitting cushions or by using a small platform under the chair. The work object can also be raised using a small wooden block or platform.

Varying the horizontal position of the chair relative to the work surface or desk may also be important. Leg and foot room should be available so the body can be moved in close to the work surface when desirable. Chairs with wheels provide a means to make repeated minor changes of position in this plane. They are a little less stable for those who must get in and out of the chair frequently, so the decision whether to use a wheeled chair must be based on the task.

Typewriting from dictation can be done more comfortably from earphones. If typing must be taken from script or printed material, the material is best mounted on a rack above the type-writer or a nearby elevated holding device rather than flat on the desk.

Drawing or handwriting is done with less neck stress if the surface is elevated at an angle with the desk. Such elevated draw-ing surfaces are in common use among artists and draftsmen but should be used more by those who do a lot of handwriting or handfiguring.

Those who read at a desk should also have available means to elevate the reading material in a rack. Devices are available that allow variation of the height and the angle at which the material is held. For those who read a great deal, investing in such reading racks is worthwhile. For more occasional readers, the same effect can be achieved using improvised props for the book or a simple desk book holder.

The problem created by sitting work is either the need for too much extension, as in looking up into the distance to a blackboard, or too much flexion, as in working down and close at a desk. The neck bends at several segments to place the head in position to do either of these things. You may tuck the chin in so that the upper neck is bent forward or leave the chin out and bend the lower neck forward. Once you obtain the feel of moving the neck at different segments, you can choose to vary the way the needed posture is achieved, and thereby spread the stresses around a little. Movement into various positions with occasional breaks to take the neck and shoulder blades through the full range of movements is essential.

There is no one "right" posture to which you should rigidly adhere all the time. The common problem for most neck and shoulder pain sufferers is that the head is held out forward from the body with the shoulders rolled forward. Repeated emphasis to avoid that particular posture is required because it is habitually overdone. That is not to say, however, that you should never go into those positions or that you should rigidly maintain the opposite posture at all times.

Two activities are so often associated with neck pain from sitting that they require special mention. One is work as a secretary–typist. The other is driving.

Many secretaries suffer pain in the muscles of the back of the neck, very often accompanied by pain and a tender spot along the inside edge of one or both shoulder blades. The prolonged position of leaning forward with the arms out in front for typing leads to fatigue of these muscles. Pressure of work overload, tensions among personalities at work, or emotional tension over personal problems all may contribute, as may muscle weakness, stiffness, and easy fatigability from inadequate exercise or poor rest and nutrition habits.

Talking on the telephone may create problems, especially when you are writing at the same time. Holding the phone receiver cradled between the head and the shoulder is stressful to the neck. This may be avoided by holding the receiver in the hand with the neck in proper posture, using a shoulder support device to cradle the receiver, or using a receiver that does not have to be held to the ear.

The neck pain problems of secretaries are not different than those of others, just more frequent. They are remedied by the same techniques discussed throughout this manual.

DRIVING

Automobile driving requires a fairly rigid position of the head and close attention. Those who drive a lot often don't realize how much effort they are making while driving. Drivers have very little freedom to move the head around.

Drivers have a marked tendency to lean the head forward to thrust the eyes closer to the windshield and thus closer to the road. This is the attitude of alertness and attention to visual detail. Good drivers never feel they can see enough and are constantly straining to look for the unexpected or the unseen.

No one should advocate a relaxed attitude while driving. All of that attention and alertness is for a good reason and should be maintained when actually driving. The driver should be aware of this straining though, so breaks can be taken when it is safe.

At every red light or other safe opportunity, the neck should be taken through a full range of motion. Long trips should be punctuated every hour by getting out of the car to stretch for a minute or two.

A very common error is to have the seat too far back from the wheel. The result is that the legs are stretched out so that the lower back is slumped and the head and neck thrust forward. The feeling of being back from the action results in more stimulus to thrust the head and shoulders forward. The seat should be up close so the knees are bent, the hips back, and the lower back in its comfortable, normal lordosis position. The shoulder blades should be pinched together. With the seat up close, shoulder blades are held comfortably in that position by contact with the seat back.

If the steering wheel is adjustable it should be kept low and close in to the body. This prevents the need to strain the neck to see over or around the wheel. It also allows the arms to rest near their normal resting position so the shoulders don't have to roll forward to place the arms out in front of the body. If the steering wheel is high and not adjustable, the driver does best to grasp it low when that can be safely done.

Mirrors should be large, clean, and well-adjusted. Inside and both right and left outside mirrors should be checked before operating the vehicle and should be used habitually. If it is necessary to turn backward to check a blind spot not covered by the mirrors, an effort should be made to roll the shoulders with the head and neck, distributing the stress throughout the spine instead of taking it all through the neck.

Windshields need to be kept clean. Dirty windshields or inadequate wipers produce increased tension by diminishing visibility. Sunglasses should be kept available in the vehicle for the same reason.

Seat belts and shoulder straps are absolutely necessary for driving safety. When properly adjusted, they also promote good posture and provide comfortable support.

Seat belts for children are not only crucial for their safety but provide the security needed so that the driver is not tempted to make sudden twisting movements to protect children during stops or turns. Before driving a vehicle, make sure any load, whether it be passengers or baggage, is secure so you have no temptation to make quick security adjustments while driving.

Automobile head rests vary a great deal. Very few actually function as head rests. They are meant to function as head stops to limit excessive backward extension of the head in the event of sudden acceleration as might occur when a car is struck from the rear. They will not function for their intended purpose if they fit down on the shoulders and lower curve of the neck. Head rests may produce unnecessary neck discomfort if they are adjusted too high so that they press high on the head. They should make contact at the base of the skull when the head is leaned back and should not press the head forward when the head is in the best posture for driving. At best, the head rest can serve as a "rest" for the driver at stop lights and other break times. It can serve consistently as a rest for the right front seat passenger.

SCHEDULING WORK

Doing demanding tasks in short segments is best when practical. If more than one job is to be done over a given time, it may be possible to shift, periodically, from one to another aspect of the job to avoid prolonged stress in the same position.

It may take time to accommodate to new stresses. People commonly have neck pain after driving all day on vacation when they are accustomed to driving only an hour a day. The same phenomenon occurs after many recreation or work activities. Often the activity would not have had to be off limits if the duration of the effort had been shorter on the first few attempts.

chapter four
DAILY HABITS

SLEEP

The ideal duration of sleep is an individual thing, but many individuals have trouble finding what is right for them. Chronic lack of sleep from overwork or worry certainly is unhealthy and may aggravate neck problems. On the other hand, many people who are prone to stiffness and aching muscles or joint pain have more trouble if they get too much sleep. The healthiest people sleep about seven hours, give or take an hour.

Sleep is a natural body function. It is difficult to directly regulate it. Sleep is most successfully regulated indirectly, by exercise and attention to other problems of the day that, when properly resolved, leave you free to obtain restful sleep at night.

Sleep should be "restorative." This means that once fully awake, you should feel fresh and ready to start again. That is more important than the number of hours slept. Too long or too short sleeping periods may be factors in "nonrestorative" sleeping but are not the only factors.

Sleeping pills frequently do not result in sleep throughout the sleeping period or in restorative sleep. For many people, pills have the opposite effect, leaving them unrested and "hung over." In some instances, when getting to sleep is the only problem, a sleeping pill may be helpful; or when habitual nonrestorative sleep or inability to sleep because of depression are the problem, antidepressant prescription drugs may help with the remedy.

Drugs are seldom a complete answer, and selecting the right drug may be difficult. Don't experiment with someone else's medicines or over-the-counter drugs to try to correct a sleeping problem. Consult your doctor if you think drugs have to be a part of the solution. Recognize that sleeping problems are not isolated problems. They are usually symptoms of other things that are wrong—inadequate exercise, excess medicines, alcohol or other drugs, and unresolved emotional conflicts are the most common problems.

Neck pain is usually relieved by rest in the proper position. Learning the techniques of rest, relaxation, and sleep that have been previously discussed allow you to sleep without much interference from neck pain. If you are consistently awakened in the middle of the night by neck pain or headache, in spite of proper application of these techniques, you should consult further with your doctor.

GETTING UP

No matter how long or how short your sleeping period, awaken yourself with ample time to go through your routine at a relaxed pace. A common characteristic of people who live with too much tension—unnecessary stress that makes them less productive and less able to deal with the necessary stresses—is that they get up in the morning already a little behind. They leave no time margin to accommodate any extra problem or pleasure.

Besides avoidance of psychological stress, you have a physical reason to allow yourself extra time in the mornings. More of this will be discussed in the section on anatomy. Suffice it to say here that the discs, which are the source of difficulty for many people, are a little swollen in the early morning. Taking the time to avoid excessive stress may protect some against any ill effect that could result because of this early-morning condition of the discs.

Calculate the time it takes to do all the things you need to do in the morning before your first commitment. Figure in ample time for exercise, bathing, and eating at a normal pace. Total up the time, then give yourself 10 to 15 extra minutes. If something goes wrong or something extra comes up, you have plenty of time to accommodate it. If everything goes according to schedule, you have a bonus of extra time for your pleasure or to be early for your first scheduled activity. Starting off your day a little ahead, instead of a little behind, is a hedge against stress that is worth much more than the 10 or 15 minutes of sleep given up for it.

HAIR CARE

The need to protect an elaborate hairdo may contribute to sustained tension on neck muscles. Hair styles that require careful head positioning through the sleeping period and caution to avoid contact or excessive movement through the day may seem attractive to some people, but whatever attractiveness they offer is not often worth the price the neck and shoulder muscles must pay for those who suffer from neck pain or tension headache. The same may be said for hair that is worn low over the eyes, requiring adjustment of the head position to provide clear vision.

Another special situation regarding hair care involves the use of shampoo basins, as are commonly used at professional hairdressing establishments. The contact surface of most shampoo basins is over a fairly small area across the middle of the back of the neck. The head is bent back, forcing the neck into extension over the contact edge of the basin. This combination of forces could be dangerous to people with severe spondylosis, arthritis, or other cause of instability of the neck. Those people should avoid shampoo basins altogether. People with neck pain but without reason to be insecure about the stability of the neck should use their neck muscles to avoid excessive extension over the shampoo basin and should warn the hairdresser to be gentle in the application of any downward force on the head while washing the hair.

SMOKING

You want to make it a habit throughout your day to do things that are in the best interest of your health. One of the most common things that too many people do habitually that is bad for their health is to smoke.

Nothing that modern man commonly does voluntarily is as devastating to health as smoking. The testimonials, circumstantial evidence, and statistical evidence of the harm done by tobacco smoke is overwhelming.

Smoking may aggravate neck and back pain because it causes coughing that increases disc and spinal fluid pressure. There is some statistical evidence that smokers have a greater frequency of ruptured discs than other people, perhaps because of coughing, perhaps from impaired circulation to the disc, or perhaps from some as yet unidentified link.

Besides any direct links between smoking and spinal disorders and pain, there is the important indirect effect of interference with general health and quality of life. Smoking has devastating effects on the heart, blood vessels, and lungs. Disturbance of the functions of these organs impairs the ability to exercise and to participate in many of the joys of life. Those limitations lead to increased emotional tensions, depression, joint stiffness, and muscle weakness, all of which may contribute to spinal pain.

Smoking doesn't just occasionally cause loss of life from lung cancer or heart attack in some few unlucky people. Smoking impairs everyone. Your health, the quality of your life, and your ability to conquer other problems, like neck pain, will be improved if you do not smoke.

HEALTHY DAYS

Make good health practices a routine part of your entire day. Include the techniques of body mechanics. Do scapula pinches, neck and shoulder stretches, and relaxation exercises at free moments through your day. Keep the attitude that you are in charge of your health and that you are not going to allow yourself to do things that will be detrimental to your health or allow unnecessary interference with the things that will benefit you.

chapter five
PSYCHOLOGICAL FACTORS

Headache is perhaps the most widely accepted physical sign of emotional tension. Though there may be many physical reasons for headache, almost everyone recognizes that headaches commonly result from fatigue, frustration, anger, or anxiety. The mechanism by which these emotional factors result in headache frequently involves tension through the neck and shoulder muscles.

In some instances, the emotional aspects of a neck pain or headache problem are the most important factors. In other cases, they are not the starting factors or the major factors, but they always play some part. Even conditions with predictable amounts of physical disturbance, such as elective surgical procedures, will result in a wide variation in pain response in the same individual, depending upon psychological factors. Anxiety, tension or depression always make head and neck pain worse, regardless of the pain.

PAIN—IS IT ALL IN THE HEAD?

Many people worry that someone else thinks their pain is "all in the mind," or they may wonder if such a thing might be true about themselves. The very nature of the question reveals a misunderstanding about pain.

Pain is not some thing "out there." There is no such substance as pain. Pain cannot be poured on or stuck in from the outside, nor can pain be cut out by the surgeon.

The body contains nerve endings which may be stimulated in various ways by various substances or events. Stimulation of those nerve endings starts a message that is relayed along nerves, across nerve cells, and across nerve connections until it reaches the part of the brain that interprets the message as a conscious thought.

Whether that message ever arrives and actually stimulates conscious awareness depends upon how many similar messages are sent at the same time, how well those messages cross the nerve connections and travel along the nerves, and how responsive the nerve cells are to those messages.

Whether the messages, once received, are interpreted as "pain" depends upon all those factors and upon the mind's interpretation of what the signal means.

Therefore, a great many factors are involved in the experience of pain other than simply what the stimulus is and what else is going on in the mind.

Pain is not always something bad. In fact, it is usually a helpful warning that something is being done wrong, something that could be harmful to the body.

Pain could be thought of as a smoke alarm system meant to protect a building. If a fire occurs, the alarm goes off and an effort is made to put out the fire. That's how it should work.

Sometimes, however, the system may be too sensitive. Every harmless bit of dust or cigarette smoke may set the alarm off, resulting in unnecessary and harmful reactions.

People who have pain for a long time may have changes occur that make the system too sensitive. Too many messages get through. Messages from harmless stimuli are interpreted as harmful.

The body has natural protective mechanisms that keep the system from being too sensitive. These may be reduced by taking pain-relieving and tranquilizing drugs and by failing to get enough exercise. This is part of the explanation for the failure of drugs to manage chronic pain, the increase in pain when drugs are withdrawn, and the success of exercise in combating these problems.

The mechanism may also be too sensitive if the mind is troubled by other factors causing anxiety or depression. The mind may be conditioned by life's circumstances to be too responsive to stimuli or to misinterpret stimuli.

The mind is occupied by many stimuli and has the capacity to interpret them in different ways. The context in which the mind receives stimuli that may be interpreted as pain can be varied by changing life circumstances and by volitional changes of mental attitudes. Simple examples are the lack of awareness of otherwise very painful injuries by athletes during competition or soldiers in battle.

The question of whether pain is all in the mind must, therefore, always be answered "yes." This does not mean that pain is "made up" in a simple, conscious way. All pains, even those from very obvious external causes such as cuts or burns are "in the mind"—only the stimuli that affect the nerve endings are "out there." The pain that is in the mind depends on those stimuli, all the nerve hookups and relays, and the attitude the mind has when the message reaches the part of the brain that can bring the stimuli to consciousness.

MIDDLE-AGE LIVES–MIDDLE-AGE NECKS

For reasons discussed in the section on anatomy, changes occur in the neck during the 30s, 40s, and 50s that may cause or aggravate pain. Common muscle tension neck pain and pain related to disorders of the discs are much less common among children, adolescents, and older people.

These middle years when changes are occurring in the neck anatomy are for most people years of great psychological stress.

Housewives are burdened with the care of chidren, suffering through the problems of school and adolescence with the children and then facing the void left in their lives as the kids leave home.

Employed people face the frustrations of work that has become boring through repetition. The physical demands of some work that seemed easy in their 20s become progressively less tolerable as the strength and resilience of youth fades.

Difficult choices of compromise to the demands of family, finances, employers, and other obligations become more frequent.

Age and specialization of skills may create fewer possibilities to change jobs or locations. This may lead to insoluble needs to compromise with the demands of the present job. The company, the boss, the foreman, or the co-workers may be unpleasant to work with but impossible to avoid without leaving the security of the job.

Marriages may fail or hang together with tension and strife. Parents age and become burdensome where they once were supportive.

Friends may suffer illnesses or failures or may move away.

All of these stresses are much more common when people are in their 30s, 40s, and 50s than they were in their 20s. The middle years are the ones in which people must face the frustrations or lost hopes and dreams and yet go on supporting not only themselves but also dependent children and parents.

These are also the years when our spines start to fail us. No wonder a strong inter-relationship between neck and back pain and anxiety and depression develops.

ESCAPE

For some people, the neck or back pain becomes a means of escape. When it all becomes too much and they feel overwhelmed, the first thing to go is the spine function. Being down with neck pain may mean an escape from a job that seems intolerable. Having the pain may mean that the spouse and kids have to demand less. It may mean that less guilt is felt for not being able to keep up with it all.

ANGER

For some people, neck or back pain becomes a way of expressing anger that has not found expression elsewhere. The worker who is hurt doing a job he should not have had to do, or doing a job that he finds beneath his abilities and unappreciated, or serving a demanding and unreasonable boss, may find it easy to vent anger and frustration through pain that keeps him from working. Everyone sees examples of this psychological mechanism in themselves and others. It always hurts more and longer if we are injured doing something we didn't want to do for someone else than had we suffered the same injury doing our own thing. The teenage boy that suffers all sorts of blows without a notice on the athletic field will be very vocal in his suffering if he bumps into something while doing a chore he didn't want to do. Husbands and wives may seem sick or in pain keeping them from doing something for the other when the real reason that they don't want to do it is because they are angry.

BARREL ON THROUGH

Some people seem to find no gain at all in being afflicted with neck pain and headache. The psychological tensions of their life situation just makes everything worse. Those who get no help or relief when they are in pain may push on to maintain their normal functions. The pain may just add one more tension, making the stress that much worse.

Tension, the result of the physical and emotional stresses of life, cannot be avoided by people who must deal with life's conflicts. There are methods of dealing directly with the effects of tension. These methods involve combined physical and psychological techniques. They are described in the chapter on relaxation exercises.

FEAR

At this point, it may help to try to define a concept that recurs throughout the considerations of attempts to recover from or function in spite of neck pain. That concept is the role played by fear. People who have made some adjustments to the pain, no matter how unsuccessful, may be unwilling to try more successful methods because they fear losing what balance they have gained.

Most people who have given up work because of neck pain really want to go back to work but are afraid to because they fear neck pain or fear not being able to readjust to the job situation. Most people who have given up family responsibilities, sex, or recreation want to return to full function and would do so were it not for fear of the consequences. Fear that things could get worse stands in the way of any attempt to make things better.

A main goal of this book to help you achieve a complete understanding of your neck pain as it relates to your life is to show you the high price you pay if you do not risk getting better. Another main goal is to arm you well enough with tools for fighting the neck pain that the chances of success are good enough to overcome that fear and risk doing the things that lead to wellness.

THE COST OF DROPPING OUT

Those who do get some help or compensation because of their pain and are thus relieved from some of the stresses of their lives often do so at great expense to them. While the middle years are ones of great stress, they are also ones of great productivity and joy. The frustrations of raising children are coupled with joy, and the more you participate in child-rearing, the more will be the reward. Most people have developed some skills and maturity in their work and can call on experience or seniority in their jobs to gain more favorable circumstances. Most jobs are done better and faster by people with some experience. The rewards and satisfactions of doing a job well should be greatest for most people in the middle years. Friendships and love relationships should be more mature and giving than those of youth.

Those who drop out of the stresses of middle life because of spinal pain also drop out of full appreciation of the rewards. The long range cost of this dropout is often much greater than appreciated at first. Some of the social implications of it will be discussed later. We will deal here primarily with the psychological implications.

Regular productive work, whether it be by an outside "public" job, or home-based, self-employed, such as housewifing or farming, is necessary to the psychological health of most people. Too much of what we all see and know of as "life" is lost if we are not productive. Even if the absence from work seems to be well-tolerated at first, it seldom is in the long run. Most people who do not work become depressed or develop behavior patterns that destroy their relationships with others and rob them of joy in their lives.

FANNING THE FIRE

The gain that is obtained by absences from work or withdrawal from home responsibility or from obligations in personal relationships may seem very nice at first. Neck pain as a mechanism to make those gains may seem very easy. However, a habit pattern can develop. Less and less pain may be used to gain more and more escape. The effect can almost be like using drugs or alcohol to escape from problems. What seems harmless enough at first may become very destructive.

The use of drugs and alcohol as a comparison is particularly meaningful for reasons beyond just demonstrating how addictions and dependency develop. Sometimes drugs, medicines, or alcohol can become the primary problem. To justify taking more pills or another drink, you must have more pain. The confusion between the need for drugs or a drink and the neck pain may become great enough that the pain comes in response to the need for alcohol or medicines.

Linking neck pain to escape from stress leads to the development of patterns of behavior. Employers, co-workers, family, and friends who were very glad to be helpful at first become less tolerant of compromises they have to make because of another's pain. This means that to go on getting those rewards, the pain must be exaggerated more and more. This exaggeration may be made not only to those directly involved, but also to doctors, leading to more and more tests and treatments.

Very few people ever enter this sort of cycle intentionally. No one who sees the full picture of it and the end result ever would. No amount of escape from problems or financial or other reward is worth what this does to people.

People enter this pattern barely aware, or sometimes totally unaware, of what they are doing. They may get encouraged in it by well-meaning friends, spouses, union advisors, attorneys, or medical practitioners. Very few people ever get into this cycle because it "is all in their head." Almost all really do have something wrong with their spines. Frequently, the problem with the anatomy of the neck is a very serious one—one that really does require some treatment or compromise of function. The problem is that as people get caught in this spiral, the treatments and the compromises can become much more devastating than the disease.

RECOGNITION

The first step in relieving the psychological aspect of a neck problem is to fully recognize it. Many times, just taking an honest look at the possibilities will make people aware of these factors. It is frequently difficult to look objectively at these possibilities. People are fearful of the inference that the pain is "all in the head" or that they have "mental problems." Both of these inferences are inaccurate oversimplifications of the problem and should not prevent an honest look at the situation.

KEEP A LOG

It may help to see these relationships by keeping a careful diary. This may be too time consuming to do for a long period but important information can often be realized in two or three weeks of careful diary keeping. The diary should include all the times you experience neck pain. The intensity and duration of the pain should be recorded. There should also be a careful, honest log of all things that bother you. Be picky and include every little thing, even things that don't seem to matter very much. Many times, the cumulative effects of repeated little irritations that you dismiss because you think they "shouldn't" bother you add up to a major annoyance and tension builder. The value of the diary is that you can see the effect of these things and their correlation with neck pain over a period of a week or more. Often patterns emerge which are not apparent when you face the stresses of life one by one and hour by hour.

OPEN UP

You need to have honest talks with the people to whom you are the closest. You need to know from your spouse, your kids, your boss, your co-workers, and your friends where you really stand with them. You need to make them be honest with you about it. You need to know how your neck pain and headaches have affected them and how it might affect your relationship with them in the future. They need to know from you what you think of them and what your intentions are. You need to talk out problems and frustrations you have with these people. You may not be able to work out all the differences to your advantage, but you must be open about your feelings. The differences need to be understood. Your neck pain cannot be a way of communicating those differences or of gaining an advantage, if you are to rid yourself of that pain and the tensions that aggravate it.

PLAN YOUR ATTACK

Once you are able to honestly evaluate the role that emotions and behavior are playing in yourself and the true feelings and expectations of others, you are in a position to make decisions about dealing with the problem. Not all of these problems are soluble. Some are, and you must identify the ones that are and put your time and energy into the solutions of them. Those that are not, you must relax about. If you are making an effort to deal with what can be dealt with and you can share your feelings about what can't be dealt with in an open, honest way, you will have lots of support. Everyone has weaknesses and problems. People look for others willing to share problems and laugh at them or talk them out.

People don't like to be manipulated by others who are not willing to face the real issues honestly. Most people with chronic pain problems feel loneliness and isolation because others have withdrawn from them. That withdrawal is usually the result of a feeling of being manipulated, from feeling that too much is being asked. People with chronic pain who don't confuse their problems of the painful condition with other psychological needs and who bear their pains without making unnecessary or excessive demands on others do not suffer that isolation. This is another example of how the long-range effects of what seems a simple, workable mechanism can be devastating. The need to manipulate for a small advantage in dealing with someone can gradually increase, eventually producing an isolation and psychological (if not physical) withdrawal of those that were close, having devastating effects on the quality of life.

Pain can become a way of life. A certain amount of advantage in dealing with employers, social agencies, family, and friends can be gained by pain-related behavior. Those who see the whole picture know that whatever the advantages, they are never worth the price that ends up being paid.

Once the psychological factors are recognized and attempts are made to deal with them honestly and to confront them, you need to set about trying to modify pain-induced behavior.

People who have accepted the "pain way of life" build all sorts of habit patterns dependent on pain. Frequently, their spouses or those they work or live with become involved in this system. All sorts of little rewards are given for pain-related behavior. Pills with a pleasant psychological side effect or a drink of alcohol is taken when the pain is bad. Anxiety-provoking social contacts are avoided when the pain is bad. And on, and on . . . Once recognized, these "pain games" must be changed to "wellness games." Deny yourself a drink or a dessert when the pain is there and reward yourself with one when you have done a hard day's work or have accomplished something that you had previously been afraid to try. Talk frankly with those close to you and get them to stop "doing you favors" when you are having pain and to reward you with some when you are not. Recognize the signals you give that ask for help or isolation—moans, sighs, grimaces, and holding the sore place. Try to stop them and ask those around you to ignore them.

TALK TO YOURSELF

Make a list of "state-of-mind commandments" that are especially meaningful to you. Write them out on a little card or piece of paper you can carry with you to read over frequently until you know them. Choose what is most fitting to you and add some of your own. The following are some examples:

I am in charge of my own health.

I am polite but open and honest about my feelings.

I treat everyone with respect, including my spouse and children.

I talk out my problems with people I am close to.

I don't let pain stop me from doing things that are important to my life.

I choose to be healthy.

I can only be in one place at a time.

I do my best now and don't worry about what might go wrong.

I believe that being strong and healthy is better than being weak and sick.

I do not let my pain be someone's problem.

I am not perfect but I am a good person.

I am getting better.

I do not depend on drugs, alcohol, or nicotine.

GUIDED IMAGERY

The above suggestions about "talking to yourself," while useful for almost everyone, may be a little simplistic and old knowledge to some people. For those who want to take this a step further, the technique of "guided imagery" is a more complex and sophisticated effort to reeducate the mind's perception of pain and the life context into which it falls.

We all recognize that the brain can directly and consciously dictate "voluntary" activity so that when the brain says "walk," the appropriate leg muscles act and walking results. Sometimes the brain does not act in such concrete, verbal terms. It reacts in response to images. Watching an erotic dance may produce physical changes of sexual excitement, watching a sad movie may make us cry, and watching someone eat when we are hungry may make us salivate.

When the mind must deal with pain, we know it is not always successful with a direct verbal approach. Telling the pain to go away or telling yourself it isn't there may help a little, but often it won't help much. One of the problems is that pain isn't really out there to take hold of or be spoken to directly. The attempts by many people to understand their pain in anatomic or medical terminology don't really lead to their being able to directly deal with pain more effectively.

Many people, only half seriously, describe their pains in terms of "burning pokers," "stabbing knives," or "bands around my head." Such terms are the language of imagery—the characterization of an abstract situation like pain by a visual image. Guided imagery is a technique that seeks to encourage the development of such an image and then attempt to gain mastery over the pain by using the terms of the image.

First practice the technique of forming a visual image. Practice with a picture or furniture object at home. Close your eyes and make a mental image of it. Then open your eyes and inspect it. Discover details your first image had left out. Do this repeatedly until your image becomes very rich in detail.

Next adopt the rest position or one of the postures described in the section on relaxation exercises. Close your eyes and imagine yourself sitting or lying in some place with which you are very familiar and in which you feel very safe. Form the image of that place in great detail.

You will next allow an image of the pain or the disorder with which you associate the pain to appear before you. This may be something very lifelike and representational, like a tightening band around the head, or it may be something very abstracted or fragmented, such as a color or a jagged line.

Relax and let it come. Once it comes, let it evolve and change a bit. Examine it in all its details. Look on every side of it. Observe its color, its texture, its form, its temperature, its smell, its sounds, its movements—everything about it. Relax and examine it without fear and without attraction or revulsion. Just examine this image of your pain very carefully.

Next begin to ask the image to change in a favorable way. Make it change so that it is less threatening. Allow it to change slowly, to transform into something more manageable. If it is a hot poker, let cool sprinkles of water gradually cool it; if it is a jagged red lightening bolt, let its corners and its point smooth and its color fade into lavender then blue; if it is a great rock upon your shoulders, let it crumble slowly away.

Once the image has evolved to something manageable and less threatening, then let it fade to gray and disappear, let the familiar safe place image return, then open your eyes, stretch, and go on about your day.

Repeating this exercise of guided imagery may allow you to get in touch with your disorder and your pain in terms that are more understandable to and manageable by your mind. It also gives you the sense of being more in control of your own well-being.

YOU ARE NOT ALONE—JUST GET MOVING

Everyone has psychological and behavior problems; everyone can do better with them than they do. Simple recognition of those facts and applied effort will start you in the right direction toward the solution of those problems. If the problems seem overwhelming and you can make no headway with them, consultation with a clergyman, psychologist, or psychiatrist may help get you over the difficulty. For most people who can recognize the difficulty and begin to work on it, professional help is not necessary. Like with exercise, the important thing is to begin moving in the right direction. Progress may be slow and, at times, difficult, but continued movement in the right direction will begin to show positive results with long-range benefits.

chapter six
DRUGS AND ALCOHOL

Although alcohol is available without prescription and not generally considered a medical drug, its use in relieving neck pain and headache is so common, and the problems associated with it so similar to those associated with prescription drugs used for the same purposes, that they will be discussed together.

Opinions about the effects of drugs vary considerably even among experts. Those given here are from the perception of the physician dealing with spinal pain. The drugs named are common examples; they are not meant to be a complete list. Specific information about drugs may be obtained from drug information centers or from your doctor or pharmacist.

Recent media attention has been given to the withdrawal of an anti-inflammatory drug, Oraflex, and a nonnarcotic analgesic, Zomax, from the American market after reports of deaths from taking these drugs. Both of these drugs had been extensively tested prior to their release. These events testify to the changeable and uncertain nature of drug usage recommendations. No doubt other drugs, perhaps some discussed in this chapter, will be condemned in the future. It would be a great disservice to those who are truly benefited by drug treatments to recommend that no drugs be taken, but these occurences underscore the need for informed discretion in the use of any medication.

ANTI-INFLAMMATORY MEDICINES

There are a large number of anti-inflammatory drugs. There are two groups—the steroidal or cortisone-like drugs, and the nonsteroidal ones that are chemically and biologically unlike cortisone.

Few neck patients take cortisone over a long period of time. Cortisone shots or short courses of cortisone are reasonably low-risk treatments that, when properly given by a physician, can help control acute symptoms of inflammation. Prolonged taking of cortisone is associated with predictable and severe side effects and must be done only for specific indication under the careful monitoring of a physician.

The nonsteroidal, anti-inflammatory drugs are a group of drugs that are chemically unlike one another and both chemically and biologically unlike cortisone. They share the characteristics of helping to reduce inflammation in joints and connective tissues and of being fairly free of effects on mental status and danger of addiction. Aspirin is the classic example. Acetaminophen (Tylenol, Datril) is not included in this group. Phenylbutazone (Butazolidin, Azolid), oxyphenbutazone (Tandearil), sulindac (Clinoril), indomethacin (Indocin), meclofenamate (Meclomen), ibuprofen (Motrin, Rufen), fenoprofen (Nalfon), naproxen (Naprosyn), tolmetin (Tolectin), diflunisal (Dolobid), and piroxican (Feldene) are commonly prescribed members of this group. Colchicine, a drug commonly used to relieve inflammation caused by gout, is also sometimes prescribed to control inflammatory responses to spinal disorders other than gout. Except for aspirin and colchicine, these drugs share the characteristics of being fairly expensive. They are all associated with potentially serious side effects, though for those who are helped by them, the risk is acceptably low to warrant long-term use. Many people are not helped by these drugs or have side effects such as stomach upset which make them intolerant of these drugs. Of course, those people should not take them.

Aspirin, because of its effectiveness, relative inexpensiveness and availability, and long-term, widespread usage is still the most popular of these drugs. It may not always be the most effective or best tolerated for a given individual, however. To make it more tolerable, a large number of coated and chemically altered forms are available, some commonly used ones being Ascriptin, Arthropan, Bufferin, Ecotrin, Trilisate, and various brands of sodium salicylate, magnesium salicylate, and sodium thiosalicylate.

MUSCLE RELAXANTS

The group of drugs termed "muscle relaxants" is, chemically, an oddly diverse group of drugs that are frequently prescribed in combined forms with common anti-inflammatories and pain relievers. Pharmacologically, it is doubtful that these drugs really have a primary effect of relaxing muscles, and clinically there seems to be little difference in the response of people with pain to these drugs from the response to the non-narcotic analgesics. Whether these drugs have any primary effect of muscle relaxation or the muscle relaxation achieved just occurs in response to the pain relief or sedative effects of these medications, the term "muscle relaxants" is generally understood by those who deal with these problems to mean a group of non-narcotic drugs of generally low addiction and side effect potential that may provide some relief from musculoskeletal pain. The effect and the precautions in use are essentially the same as for the anti-inflammatories and non-narcotic pain relievers. Treating this as a distinct class of drugs makes little sense from a clinical point of view, but common use and the influence of promotional advertising perpetuates the practice.

Commonly used examples, including the combination forms, are chlorphenesin (Maolate), orphendrine (Norflex, Norgesic), chlorozoxone (Paraflex, Parafon), methocarbamol (Robaxin, Robaxisal), metaxolone (Skelaxin), and carisoprodol (Soma, Soma Compound).

Cyclobenzaprine (Flexeril) is chemically and therapeutically so similar to the tricyclic group of drugs considered under antidepressants that it is best considered in that discussion.

Another drug commonly promoted and used as a muscle relaxant is diazepam (Valium), a drug with such potent anti-anxiety effects and side effects that it, along with similar drugs, is best considered with the discussion of tranquilizers. The same may be said for meprobamate (Equanil, Miltown) which is also sometimes used for muscle relaxation.

TRANQUILIZERS

Drugs considered as tranquilizers all have the effect of altering mental status and have some addictive potential. Most drugs called tranquilizers have a "downer" effect, helping to ease anxiety and nervousness. Many of them have an effect not unlike alcohol in that they have a rapid initial calming effect and a long range danger of depression and habituation.

Few people become addicted to these drugs in the sense that addiction can develop to narcotic pain relievers. Many people, however, become habituated to them. These drugs provide what seems to be some relief for a short time, but they undermine the will and determination to get to the real problem with real solutions and except for very short-term use for acute anxiety they do little real good.

Phenobarbital is the classic example of this type of drug. Because it and other barbiturates have been used and misused for a long time, the hazards are commonly known and, thus, it is not prescribed as often as it once was. Other, newer drugs with somewhat similar effects and hazards are in very common use. The hazards, of course, depend on dose, frequency of ingestion, and number of days of use.

Meprobamate (Equanil, Miltown), hydroxyzine (Atarax, Vistaril), and the benzodiazepines (Librium, Serax, Tranxene, Ativan, Centrax, Valium) are commonly used drugs of this group. Perhaps the best known of these drugs is diazepam (Valium). Because its use became so widespread, some of the hazards of diazepam dependency have become the subject of general media discussion and, thereby, popular knowledge.

Because of its widespread use to control many anxiety, pain, and tension related symptoms, diazepam (Valium) is probably the drug of this type that is most commonly abused to the detriment of neck pain and headache sufferers. The result of prolonged use is drug dependency, diminished energy and motivation, depression, and reduced pain tolerance. Diazepam deserves the criticism it has received in those regards but probably no more so than less famous drugs of the same group. All of these tranquilizing drugs have the potential to produce those same harmful side effects when taken for chronic pain. There are specific indications for the use of these drugs and they should be taken only under the management of a physician who is aware of what other medicines are being taken and what other problems are present (most particularly, the problem of controlling chronic headache, neck pain, or back pain).

ANTIDEPRESSANTS

Several drugs are used primarily to control depression. Some of these drugs have been found to be effective in the control of chronic pain. Whether the pain seems less bad as the depression is relieved, the relief of depression allows a more healthful lifestyle resulting in fewer pain producing stimuli, or whether some intermediate phase of the chain of transmission from stimulus to conscious pain perception is altered by these drugs is not completely understood. All of these modes of action may work together. Regardless, the observation made is that many people with chronic pain seem to improve after taking one of these medications for a period of time. The positive effects are not as rapid as they are with analgesic and tranquilizing medication.

Many of the antidepressant drugs that are commonly used in attempts to control pain are sometimes referred to as "tricyclics" because of the shape of the chemical representation of the basic molecule. Common examples are amitriptyline (Elavil, Amitid, Endep), doxepin (Adapin, Sinequan), amoxapine (Ascendin), nortriptyline (Aventyl, Pamelor), protryptyline (Vivactil), maprotyline (Ludiomil), desipramine (Norpramin, Pertofrane), and imipramine (Tofranil). Chemically distinct but pharmacologically similar is trazodone (Desyrel). These drugs may be prepared combined with tranquilizers (Deprol, Limbitrol, Etrafon, Triavil).

Many people experience unpleasant physical side effects from these drugs, such as dry mouth, visual blurring, and increased appetite, and unpleasant mental side effects such as bad dreams, sedation, or nervousness. There is a great deal of individual variation in response to these drugs, so the safest and most effective use of them may require careful monitoring, including blood testing, under the supervision of a physician expert in the use of them. The latter is more apt to be necessary for patients who are going to try to take the maximum tolerated dose, who are going to try to continue to take the drug in spite of side effects, or who have a major primary problem with depression.

PAIN RELIEVERS

Medicines called pain relievers vary enormously in their mode of action, effects, and dangers. Nonsteroidal anti-inflammatory drugs may effectively be used for pain relief since much musculoskeletal pain is the result of inflammation.

Acetaminophen (Tylenol, Datril) is one of the safest pain relieving medications and is available without prescription at reasonable cost. Propoxyphene (Darvon) is an intermediate-strength pain reliever with mild addictive potential and slightly greater risk of side effects. It is frequently combined with aspirin (Darvon Compound) or acetaminophen (Darvocet, Wygesic) to increase its effectiveness. Taking it with alcohol or other potent drugs may substantially increase the dangers of its use.

Ethoheptazine (Zactane) is another commonly used non-narcotic pain reliever with the same general properties as propoxyphene. It is also commonly combined with aspirin (Zactirin).

The nonsteroidal anti-inflammatory drugs have either a direct or indirect (or both) effect on relieving pain. An anti-inflammatory preparation (Motrin, Nalfon) or a chemical derivation of one (Anaprox, Ponstal) may be prescribed as a pain reliever.

Many over-the-counter and some prescription drugs used as pain relievers are really combinations of tranquilizers, anti-inflammatories, stimulants (caffeine), and pain relievers. Commonly prescribed examples include Equagesic (meprobamate, ethoheptazine, and aspirin) and Fiorinal (butalbital, aspirin, phenacetin, and caffeine), Synalgos (promethazine, aspirin, phenacetin, and caffeine), and Zactirin Compound (ethoheptazine, aspirin, phenacetin, and caffeine).

Pain relievers containing codeine have more addiction potential than the drugs discussed above. Like all narcotic drugs, they become less effective the more they are used. They have the unpleasant side effect of constipation. Codeine, too, is frequently combined with other drugs to increase its potency and decrease the dose of codeine needed for the desired effect. Aspirin (Empirin with Codeine), acetaminophen (Empracet with Codeine, Phenaphen with Codeine, Tylenol with Codeine), and multiple-ingredient combinations (Fiorinal with Codeine) are frequently designated with the following numbers: "2" meaning 15 milligrams of codeine, "3" for 30 milligrams of codeine, and "4" signifying 60 milligrams (or one grain) of codeine.

Synthetically made drugs very similar, chemically and biologically, to codeine have been developed in an attempt to provide increased effectiveness with decreased side effects. In the commonly used doses and combination forms, these drugs seem to have more addiction potential than the commonly used doses and forms of codeine. At least the number of patients with neck and back pain who have developed a harmful dependency on narcotic drugs seems to be greater with these codeine derivatives than it does with codeine itself. Oxycodone (Percodan, Percocet, Tylox) is the most commonly abused of these drugs. Hydrocodone (Vicodin) and dihydrocodeine (Synalgos DC) are other examples of this type of drug.

Pentazocine (Talwin) is an intermediate-strength narcotic drug similar in strength and potential for addiction to, but chemically unlike, the codeine drugs. It should not be used except in short-term acute pain situations.

Morphine, oxymorphone (Numorphan), hydromorphone (Dilaudid), and meperidine (Demerol, Mepergan) are strong narcotic medications that should be used for neck pain only in very unusual circumstances and, then, almost always in a hospital or very controlled situation.

ALCOHOL

Having thus considered the different types and classes of neck pain medicine, we should return to mention of alcohol. Alcohol is very commonly misused for relief of neck pain and other chronic pain conditions.

The reason people become habituated to the use of alcohol for control of pain is very similar to the reason many become habituated to the use of some of the drugs just described. The drugs most often involved in this phenomenon are alcohol, tranquilizers, and codeine derivatives. Use of these drugs together or in combination is particularly dangerous.

Patients who habitually use alcohol to relieve pain or who rely heavily on tranquilizers or codeine derivatives or some combination of these drugs have more trouble ridding themselves of neck and back pain than any other single group of patients, regardless of the anatomic origin of the pain.

If you rely heavily on alcohol with or without other drugs to control neck pain or headache, it is absolutely necessary that you free yourself of that burden if you are ever to be free of the neck pain.

For some people, the first and primary problem is alcohol or drug dependency. Some people have a constitution so that they are so susceptible to the addictive potential of alcohol or certain drugs that they must consider themselves "allergic" to them and must absolutely avoid any contact with them. Their health and, indeed, their lives depend on avoiding the alcohol or drug.

Some people already caught in the trap of such alcohol or drug dependency find that escape from neck or back pain becomes a "reason" to go on taking the drug. Others may have never been aware of their susceptibility to alcohol or drugs and only experience the difficulty after they have developed a spinal problem and begin to use alcohol or drugs for neck, head, or back pain. Once you are caught in this web of habituation, your mind's craving for the drug becomes so strong that the pain appears as a signal and justification for more drugs.

There is no escaping the cycle of neck pain and dependency on alcohol and/or addictive drugs without withdrawal from the drugs and alcohol. The idea that the drugs or alcohol will be given up as soon as something is done "to fix the neck" never works. If alcohol or drug addiction is already a problem, it needs to be discussed frankly with doctor, spouse, and those that care. Professional help is likely to be needed.

If there is only a suggestion that alcohol or drug dependency could be part of the problem, the alcohol or drug needs to be cut off immediately.

Most people can tolerate an occasional drink of alcohol without serious consequence. For those who can tolerate it, alcohol can serve as a tension reliever. When alcohol interferes with normal function and responsibilities or when it interferes with meaningful communication with loved ones, it should be avoided altogether.

For those who have neck pain, particular care must be taken to avoid using alcohol as a pain reliever. The records of those that have tried provide overwhelming evidence of the danger and lack of success of this method of neck pain and headache control.

If you have enough experience with alcohol to know that it brings you pleasures safely and without risk of making things worse for yourself, you may be able to use it to your advantage. Deprive yourself of alcohol at times you are down with neck pain—you must do that anyway to avoid the risk of using it for neck pain. Reward yourself with a drink if you are feeling well or if you have made some substantial progress in returning to a normal life.

The above endorsement of the use of alcohol is a very qualified one. No one who does not have a history of successful use of alcohol without ill effects should ever begin to use it when having any trouble with their health, including neck pain. Alcohol should not be used by anyone taking any pain-relieving or tranquilizing medicine. Alcohol should never be taken in excess. Alcohol should never be used to relieve neck pain or symptoms associated with spinal disorders. If alcohol is used at all, it should be used infrequently, in small doses, and at times when symptoms are diminished and function improved.

NATURAL PAIN RELIEVERS

There is a growing body of scientific information about hormones that the body produces to provide pain relief. There is still much to be understood about these natural pain-control hormones called endorphins.

The body seems to produce more of these pain-resisting hormones if the individual exercises vigorously on a regular basis in the way discussed in the section on general fitness.

The natural production of these hormones may be suppressed by taking pain medicines. That may explain why medicines don't help much after a while and why pain gets worse, temporarily, if regular medicines are stopped. This mechanism would explain the common observation that regular reliance on medicine to control chronic neck or back pain often only makes things worse, and why, given enough time, fitness exercise makes it better.

chapter seven
WEIGHT AND DIET

A great deal has been written about diet and health. As it relates to neck pain, the only common problem with diet that is associated with neck pain is the consumption of too many calories.

NUTRITION

To be sure, a balanced, nutritional diet is a requirement of general good health. People on extreme weight-reduction diets or people who, for some reason, do not get a balanced diet should take a multivitamin pill so they get their minimum daily requirement of vitamins each day. Women past menopause are wise to take a vitamin and mineral supplement including extra calcium to try to maintain bone strength. Other than under those situations, neck pain does not indicate a need for special diet supplements.

It is particularly useless and unfortunate for people to devote money and hopes to special diet and vitamin "cures" for neck pain and related complaints involving musculoskeletal discomfort. These "cures" represent well-meaning but misguided attempts to buy an easy way out of problems that must be attacked by learning proper care, exercise, and stress control. Unfortunately, the latter requires a lot of dedication and effort whereas the former only requires some money, popping a few pills, or some unusual diet combinations. The problem is that the dedicated effort approach really helps and fad diets and pills don't.

WHAT SHOULD YOU WEIGH?

Overweight causes increased difficulty with neck pain because of its effect on overall spinal posture and because it interferes with the general feeling of well-being and energy.

An individual's ideal weight may depend on many factors. No people, however, have neck pain because they carry too little excess fat.

Most well-conditioned athletes weigh a great deal less than their average, nonathletic counterparts, even in spite of the extra muscle development they carry. Exceptions that occur in well-publicized sports like football occur because the sports attract heavily built individuals, the athletes' degree of muscle development is extreme, and, in some cases, the athletes' excess body fat is carried intentionally. Runners, swimmers, tennis players, basketball players, and most other athletes, in contrast, weigh a good bit less than nonathletes of the same height.

The lean, conditioned (but not heavily muscled) body weight of most men of 66 to 72 inches in height is between 135 and 175 pounds. Some people may wish to carry more weight because they think it looks good or helps them in some way, but if the goal is to keep body weight and excess fat down, few men should carry more than 175 pounds.

The ideal weight for women should be adjusted down according to height and body build. The image of a lean, healthy, body build for women is more accurately portrayed by the media than is that of men. Thus, the thin look of most models and actresses more nearly approximates the ideal healthy body build for women than does the macho, heavily built image of football players for men.

What is or is not attractive about thinness and fat is certainly open to question. Many people think they and their loved ones look healthier, more robust, more successful, and happier if they carry some excess fat. Maintaining that look, however, may be a luxury that is not worth the cost for spinal pain sufferers.

If you count up all the miles you walk, stairs you climb, feet the body weight is raised and lowered getting in and out of beds, chairs, and automobiles and multiply these by the body weight that is lifted, an astounding number of foot-pounds of work can be documented. Reduction of body weight by only a few pounds, therefore, can substantially reduce the stresses that are placed on the body even by ordinary activity.

Excess abdominal fat results in a forward shift of the body's center of gravity—the central axis of the body's weight around which the spine and muscles must support the body to keep it upright. The stretched-out abdominal muscles are less able to pull the center of gravity back toward the spine to exert pressure through the abdomen to support the spine.

The only way the lumbar spine can accommodate this additional stress is to sway further—to go into more lordosis, so as to tip the upper body backward. Otherwise, the body would topple forward.

As the upper body is tipped backward, the head and shoulders are allowed to slump forward to balance the upper body and bring the eye level straight ahead.

In this way, excess abdominal fat contributes to the slouched, slumped, head-forward posture that causes so much neck, shoulder, and head pain. The extra fatigue caused by carrying that fat around further aggravates the pain.

Excess weight is not a primary cause of neck pain, and weight reduction by itself will not cure most neck pain. But weight reduction helps, and without it complete relief is less attainable.

WEIGHT REDUCTION DIET

How do you lose weight? For some people who recognize that they have been regularly eating too much, the answer is obvious.

Many overweight people honestly believe that they do not overeat, and they may have good reason to believe that. They may eat far less than thin spouses or friends. They may eat fewer calories than what is said to be right for them.

For some people, it just isn't fair. There is no answer to that, but fair or not, those people can still lose weight.

If the calorie intake is reduced enough, everyone can lose weight. Some people must reduce their intake far more than others. Some must keep it reduced for longer than others. Sometimes weight loss is unexplainably uneven with no loss at all for days or weeks, then loss for awhile, and then another plateau of no loss.

Diet pills, for some people, are either not safe, are ineffective, or are both. They have the bad effect of displacing the responsibility for weight control. They may also increase feelings of tension and anxiety. The control must come from your determination, not from a pill.

The essential features of any workable diet are that total calorie consumption must be reduced and that the diet must be acceptably safe and tolerable for permanent maintenance.

Extreme, fad diets that severely limit the choice of foods or are overloaded with certain food types while lacking others usually work, temporarily, either because they are bad nutrition or because they are so unpalatable that the real effect is to drastically reduce calorie intake.

Certain popular diets that are careful to provide good nutrition and then have a built-in mechanism to guide the dieter to a permanent maintenance diet that is palatable and nutritious are acceptable. The enthusiasm generated by their proponents and the opportunity to go on them with someone are big plus factors to help get started.

Diets that promise to take several pounds off very rapidly may have an appeal—but that is the wrong appeal. If you are overweight, you have probably been so for a long, long time and you have probably gradually gotten more so. What you want is to reverse that direction—permanently—to begin losing instead of gaining and to keep losing until you reach a lean body build and then to stay there, never to go back in the direction of gaining again.

You want a diet that promises you only that—adequate nutrition and a permanent change from the direction of gaining to that of losing and then maintenance without ever changing back to the direction of gaining again. You don't care how fast you get there as long as you keep going in the right direction.

Those are the important principles. Accept them, even

though it isn't fair that you don't lose weight in spite of a reasonably low calorie intake. If the calorie intake is low enough for long enough, you will lose weight. Accept that the diet change must provide adequate nutrition, that it must be palatable, and that it must be permanent. If you adhere to those principles, you will succeed. Beyond that commitment, there are a number of safe "tricks" to make adherence to those principles easier.

UNDERSTANDING HUNGER

Analysis of what makes you want to eat may help establish a diet pattern you can live with. Most people assume they eat because they are hungry and that the hunger is their body's way of telling them they need more nutrition. In fact, it is a rare instance when most people in developed nations are in any real nutritional need for more calories. As successful dieters and athletes on high-energy-expenditure, low-calorie-intake regimens find, the real nutritional needs of our body are a great deal less than what most people consume. That is why even a quite substantial reduction in calorie intake will often not lead to weight loss. If the number of calories is reduced enough for long enough, however, weight will always come off.

If we don't eat for nutritional need, then why do we get hungry? Of course, food tastes and smells good and partaking of it is one of life's great pleasures. But many of the people who enjoy that pleasure most don't eat too much. Most people who do overeat recognize that they eat too fast or too much to be really savoring the taste and smells.

The consumption of food is associated from the first moments of life with comfort and attention. Little wonder that when we feel depressed, lonely, bored, or frustrated one of the first things we feel is hunger and one of the first places we turn to is the refrigerator. Eating seldom helps for more than a few minutes, though, and for those who are overweight, the guilt feelings that follow often just make the depression and frustration greater.

Many people eat when they are angry. Anger with a spouse, kids, boss, or loved one that is not expressed directly sometimes results in frustrations that lead to diet abuse. Many people do things to damage themselves when they are angered by someone else, and one of the most popular ways to accomplish that is over-eating.

Many people eat in response to these emotions from habit. Few people consciously think, "I am angry, therefore I will eat," or "I am bored, therefore I will eat." Most people who eat for these reasons do it mostly from an unconscious, repeated pattern of behavior.

You may be able to recognize the things that make you hungry by keeping a list for a few days of exactly what you eat and when and what you are doing and feeling at the time you eat. Patterns may emerge that help you see better why you are eating than you could ever see by trying to figure it out one snack at a time.

Many people discover when they make such a list that they have been eating a great deal more than they realized. Another thing that sometimes happens is that making the list becomes part of the cure—if you know you have to confess to it by writing it down, you may decide eating is not really worth it and pass it up.

EFFECTS OF EXERCISE ON WEIGHT

Combining exercise with diet is a popular and valid approach to weight control. However, many misconceptions exist about the role of exercise and weight control. Many people say they should lose weight because of the amount of exercise they get while working or that they have to eat "well" because they get so much exercise or do so much work.

In fact, losing weight by exercise alone is almost impossible. Only very extreme amounts of exercise such as that obtained by long-distance runners running 50 or more miles a week ever seem to have a substantial direct effect on weight. Even then, the contribution of exercise is only partial, because the thinness those people maintain is, in part, due to the fact they usually consume fewer calories than people who are less physically active. Contrary to what many people think, these people who get extreme amounts of exercise usually have smaller appetites than other people and smaller appetites than they themselves have when they are not exercising so vigorously.

Exercise or physical work can even have a detrimental effect on weight control if it is used as an excuse to go off the diet. The actual calories burned by exercise may contribute only a small part of the benefit.

Regular exercise requires a reordering of the day's activities that helps remove the temptation to eat. During the hours before exercise, eating is undesirable because it causes abdominal cramping, discomfort, or nausea while exercising. Most people do not feel like eating right after exercise.

It may be best to purposely schedule your exercise at times you would be most tempted to go off your diet.

People who exercise regularly feel healthy and strong and do not want to abuse their bodies by diet abuse.

Exercise usually improves regular bowel function, relieving the tendency some people have to overeat or snack because of vague feelings of stomach or abdominal discomfort.

Many people eat because they are depressed, bored, frustrated, or angry. While some of those problems may require more direct attack on the source of the trouble, it is better to release the frustration through a healthful displacement activity, such as exercise, than it is through an unhealthful one such as snacking or overeating.

DIET HINTS

Besides coordination of your diet with exercise, a number of other helpful and harmless tips can make for successful or at least less painful dieting:

- Drink lots of water, especially a glass or two just before meals.
- Never eat anything except at regular meals.
- Don't snack while watching television or reading. If you watch television a lot, try knitting or wood carving to keep hands busy at the same time.
- Try to get maximum enjoyment from what you do eat. Take small bites. Eat slowly. Concentrate on the taste and smell.

- Don't read, watch television or have family arguments while eating.
- Put only one piece of food in your mouth at a time.
- Put the knife and fork completely down and totally empty the mouth before picking them up again.
- Don't talk about your diet, especially at meal time.
- Many people, especially housewives, can't stand to see food wasted and will act as the garbage disposal for what kids leave on their plates. Give it to the dog or get used to throwing it away—never put it in your mouth.
- Use skimmed milk, whipped margarine, diet beverages, and broiled or baked rather than fried meats.
- Avoid simple sugars. Foods with high sugar content, such as candies and soft drinks, cause more problems than just their calorie content. They cause rapid up-and-down swings in blood sugar. Not long after taking them, a "down" feeling occurs that can be relieved (only for a short time) by taking more sugared food. A cycle develops of craving more and more sugar-foods. A diet high in calories and low in nutrition results. Kids can get by without cookies and soft drinks, especially if keeping the stuff out of the house helps keep Mom or Dad healthy.
- Stay away from fast food restaurants. If you can't, find ones with a salad bar and eat only salad and unsugared drinks.
- Assign yourself something to do other than eat every time that hunger for a snack occurs. Exercise is the most healthful thing and will often work to dispel the hunger.

KEEPING IT OFF

Most people who are overweight have been "on" lots of diets and already know these and other hints very well. What is wrong is that anytime you go "on" a diet, there is an implication that someday you will go "off" of it and when you do, you will likely gain back whatever you lost and then some.

What is needed is a permanent change of diet, a change of what you eat and why you eat. You must eat for adequate nutrition and for the enjoyment of the food in limited amounts. You cannot eat to resolve anger, frustration, or vague feelings of discontent, or for more than basic nutritional needs. No matter how low the calorie intake has to go to keep you lean, that is where it must be—even if that is not fair compared to other people.

You will find that a successful diet and a slim physique is its own reward. But give yourself a little extra—put aside the money you would have spent on what you didn't eat, make a bet with your spouse, or have a contest with someone else who needs to lose, so that as you reach milestones in attaining your goal, you will get little extra awards.

chapter eight
SEX

Headache, usually neck-tension related, is the classical reason given by a marriage partner for not wanting to have sexual intercourse. The sometimes-related symptom of low back pain is second.

Many of the reasons that headache, neck pain, and back pain might be associated with avoidance of sexual activity have already been touched upon in this text, but, since it is such an important part of life for so many people and such a commonly stated problem with neck and back pain sufferers, it will be worth some repetition.

TRUE SEX-RELATED HEADACHE— AN UNUSUAL PHENOMENON

Most people who have headaches at times that they might be expected to engage in sexual activity or during sexual activity do so for reasons related to psychological and social factors associated with sex-related tension. Most of this chapter will deal with that type of sex-related headache because it is exceedingly common. A very rare type of headache so called "orgasmic headache" or "benign coital cephalgia" (medical jargon for headache during sex) needs some mention because, although very uncommon, the subject and dramatic nature of it arouse the interest of the media, so many people have heard of and wonder about it.

It is no surprise that sexual arousal and especially orgasm are related to certain abrupt changes in physical functions. Breathing is faster, pulse is rapid, blood pressure increases, sweating increases, and muscles tense. Some few people have an unusual sensitivity of the blood vessels of the brain to such changes. This may result in the very abrupt onset of a severe headache at the time of sexual excitement. The pain may be severe enough to warrant a trip to the emergency room when it first occurs. The duration is usually quite brief.

Such sudden changes in the blood vessels of the brain are similar to those that occur in classical migraine headaches and in some people who are thought to have common migraine headaches. The drugs that control or prevent migraine headaches can usually be used to effectively prevent orgasmic headache.

Well less than one percent of instances of sex-avoidance or compromise in sexual activity because of head and neck pain is related to true vascular, orgasmic headache. The very abrupt onset at the height of sexual excitement, extreme severity of the pain, and rapid improvement are quite distinct from the prolonged dull, aching, tight, pressured feeling of the muscle tension headache that is so common. If you are uncertain about distinguishing the type of headache and neck pain, a visit to a neurologist or an internist or family physician who treats headaches should make the diagnosis more certain.

BODY MECHANICS OF SEX

To be sure, certain positions and movements commonly used in the sex act can be physically stressful to the back and neck. Forceful hyperextension of the lumbar spine as the man might do in the male-on-top, conventional intercourse position could be painful in some back conditions. Any extreme or unusual posture might become exaggerated to the point of causing back or neck pain during the passion of sexual activity.

The same position and movement recommendations that were given in the chapters on posture, body mechanics, and exercise apply to sex as they would to any other activity. The muscle tension associated with sexual activity and excitement may add some increased stress to the neck. Extreme positions of the neck should be avoided. A position should be selected that is not likely to lead to excessive stressful neck posture at the height of sexual excitement. Proper use of pillows can further safeguard against such a possibility.

OTHER CAUSES OF PAIN FROM SEX

Most people find that sexual excitement relieves them from other pains and tensions. Many people find that sleep comes easily after sexual activity.

If sex can release people from tension and pain and allow them to relax, and if sex can be accomplished safely by those with neck and back pain, why then is pain from sex or avoidance of sex such a common complaint among neck and back pain sufferers? To answer that question, we must leave the consideration of the spine as an anatomic structure and return to a look at the full picture of the people and the stresses that are upon them.

Remember that spinal structures often begin to fail when people hit their 30s, 40s, and 50s—times of many stresses and frustrations. This is also a time of difficult sexual adjustment.

The sexual desire of earlier years is linked, in part, to desire for reproduction. Once enough children have been born, fear of additional unwanted pregnancies may lead to the desire to avoid sex or fear of sex. For those who have not been able to have children, have had difficult pregnancies or gynecologic problems, or have had unsuccessful marriages, the anxieties of those situations may be associated with sex, leading to avoidance or fear of sex.

The romance of early relationships pales with familiarity and repetition and is diluted in importance by worries about kids, jobs, and finances. With the loss of romance, the feeling of sexual attractiveness diminishes and with it, the desire for sex. People who don't feel sexually attractive don't want sex, just like people who don't feel like they are good at a job or a sport don't want to engage in it.

In middle age, people often gain weight, lose muscle power and tone, get wrinkles in their skin, and otherwise show signs of aging. Television, magazines, and movies portray a certain image of what is supposed to be sexually attractive. As the changes of middle age occur, people are less and less able to copy these images the media sets for sexual attractiveness. As we become less like what is supposed to be sexy, we become more afraid and reluctant about our own sexuality.

Many are burdened with the demands of financial obligation, caught in jobs where they don't have the power they would like to have, and, seeing their physical strength and resilience diminish, often have some problems with consistent sexual function.

Sex may be the dominant force in the lives of young, energetic people who want to reproduce and are less burdened with the stresses of middle age. As sex becomes a less dominant force, the enjoyment and successful performance of the sex act often diminishes or becomes inconsistent.

Most men past 30 experience occasional loss of sexual power—become unable to obtain or hold an erection during attempts at sexual intercourse. These are normal occurrences. They are often frightening to men, making them feel inadequate or powerless. They may make women feel undesired. These normal occurrences should not have the psychological effects that they do. The most common reason for repeated occurrences of sexual impotence is the fear of its occurrence. The anxiety associated with the fear that impotence will happen again makes its happening again much more likely.

Sexual participation has always been a way in which people show love and appreciation for each other. Unfortunately, the reverse is true also—denial of sexual participation has always been a way for people to express anger and disappointment to one another.

If one partner finds it difficult to say, "I'm angry with you," what is said instead (by action if not by words) is, "I won't have sex with you," or if they have the need to cover up the true feelings even more, "I won't have sex with you because I have a headache."

So neck pain as a reason for not having sex can help avoid the fears of pregnancy, avoid the fears of unsatisfactory sexual performance, avoid unpleasant memories that may have become associated with sex, avoid verbally expressing disappointment and anger that is hard to express, and can work in many like ways to fulfill some psychological need of the moment.

Pains and illnesses such as headache and back pain may be used for this purpose, especially at a time of life when sexual desire may have decreased some anyway because of feelings of lost romance and unattractiveness, worries over other important facets of life, or feelings of powerlessness and depression.

So neck pain and headache can be used to avoid an activity that may not seem very desirable at the time, may carry some threat to the ego, and may be symbolic of giving love and affection when the dominant feeling is anger and frustration.

Headache and neck pain works for this—for the moment. But what is the price—at the moment and longer range? The person with pain suffers the loss of the release and fulfillment associated with sex. Further estrangement from the partner occurs, not only because the sexual pleasure has been denied, but because it has been denied in a way that is not totally honest. That estrangement results in more frustration, more tension, more stress—more headache. There follows a temptation to further exaggerate the incapacity caused by the head and neck pain in order to save face.

SOLVING THE PROBLEMS

What can be done? The most important part of the solution is recognizing the problem. An honest consideration of all the feelings you may have about sex and your sex partner and of all the fears you associate with performance and consequences of sex is the first step.

People need to know not only how they think and feel about these things, but also how their sex partner regards them, both as their partner is concerned, and as they are concerned.

Many people find it difficult to talk to each other about these problems. Talking to each other about them is an absolutely necessary part of the remedy. Such talk is not only necessary to the full recognition of the problem, but is a big part of the solution.

If you find it impossible to begin by talking to your partner, begin by talking to someone else. Confide in a friend. You will be surprised to find that there is nothing very unusual about these problems—most people experience them in one way or another and are glad to have someone with whom to discuss them honestly. If you are unsuccessful in that, professional counseling from clergy, marriage counselors, psychologists, or psychiatrists can help. The essential fact, though, is that the talk can't stop with a professional or a friend—it must come back to a full honest disclosure of feelings between you and your partner.

Sexual desires do wax and wane. There are times people don't feel sexy. Partners need to recognize that about each other and talk about it and be considerate with one another and make reasonable compromises without using false reasons for feelings.

Some women have good reason to fear pregnancies or pelvic disorders. Their partners need to know about these fears and be supportive in seeking medical solutions or reassurances.

Men do have times they cannot obtain or hold an erection or that they ejaculate prematurely. They need to talk about how that makes them feel and listen to their partner talk about how it makes her feel and then both need to reassure the other that these things sometimes normally occur and that a relaxed attitude about it is the best measure.

Feelings of anger and disappointment need to be talked out, not acted out through withdrawal from participation in sex or other activities of life. Talking out anger is so difficult for many people that they have long become accustomed to using other methods to vent their anger. They are not consciously aware that what they are doing is motivated by frustration and anger.

Open talk about anger and disappointment between partners can be risky. Fear of being able to control the anger or fear of the partner's reaction are major reasons that true feelings are often suppressed. These fears are almost always greater than what actually happens, though. The true feelings haven't really been suppressed, only disguised in actions that are much more damaging than words—to both partners.

chapter nine
RECREATION

People need to have fun. To deny yourself the activities of life that bring pleasure is to deprive yourself the joy of life. Pleasure, to be sure, is gained from work, sex, and interpersonal relationships, but people need some additional, occasional pleasures outside these more regular occurrences.

What people choose for recreation varies with individual choice and experience. Some activities, of course, are more strenuous to the neck than others. A few sports carry such high risks of neck injury that they are not advisable.

Sports that risk sudden violent stress to the neck are those that should be avoided. Wrestling, boxing, trampolining, tumbling, water and snow skiing, and vigorous contact sports such as football and hockey are examples. The problem with these activities is that they offer very little capacity to control the intensity or avoid the possibility of sudden injury.

Any sport that risks direct head contact or forceful bending of the neck is risky. Nothing should be done "head first." Sledding, if done at all, should be done seated. Diving head first carries particularly high risk of neck injury. It is best to avoid diving head first all together. If done at all, it must be in deep, clear water where no swimmers or other objects are in the water beneath. The head should be tucked in, not extended. Never dive in shallow water or in lakes or rivers where underwater obstructions may lurk unseen.

Many other sports have some potential for neck injury but the risk is under much greater control. If you can avoid the possibility of sudden violent stress, the other factors to consider are the intensity and the duration of effort. These two factors can be controlled in most sports at least to some degree. The greatest control is possible in the activities discussed under general fitness exercise. No other sports can be done with the benefit and degree of safety that these can, but with some intelligent compromise, you can be reasonably safe and derive enjoyment from other sports.

Racquet sports involve a lot of quick stop and go activity that can be stressful to the spine. Handball requires more twisting stress than do sports utilizing racquets or paddles. Twisting and hyper-extension of the neck in tennis is most often associated with overhead shots and serving. When first trying to return to racquet sports after a neck injury, you do best to begin with practice sessions of short duration using a backboard or with another player in a completely noncompetitive situation. Slowly increase the length of each workout and return to competitive playing and attempting overhead shots only after you have demonstrated the ability to withstand long workouts, on a noncompetitive basis, without pain.

Those with a history of difficulty caused by extension of the neck should avoid forceful overhead and serving postures that require that the neck be extended and twisted. Modifications of these strokes are possible with only small compromise of the competitive edge and great saving on neck stress.

The same principles apply to such sports as basketball, softball, and soccer. Short-duration practice sessions slowly working up to competitive intensity are necessary for a long while before you return to full effort.

Golf can usually be enjoyed by people with neck pain. Short rounds and avoidance of full-effort, full-swing strokes are in order at first. The same smoothness, head and body control, and rhythmic movement that make a good golf swing provide safety for the neck. Some people find that the need to control and smooth the swing to avoid hurting the neck actually improves their scores even if it shortens the distance of their longest drives. The principles of car riding need to be applied to golf cart riding.

Fishing, hunting, hiking, camping, and similar outdoor activities are subject to great variations in duration and intensity. Attention to the principles of good body mechanics and avoidance of stress, beyond what is accustomed, allow safe return to these activities. Planning ahead so that you are certain not to be caught in situations where lifting, carrying, or other stresses, beyond what you are conditioned for, is the most important consideration in returning to these activities.

For recreation that involves riding, duration must be tempered. Bumpy riding such as horseback, trail bike, or jeep trail riding may be quite stressful to the neck and should be approached cautiously. Even less stressful riding such as in cars, road bikes, and boats can produce neck pain if the duration of the activitiy is too long at first. Most of these enjoyable activities can be pursued, even in the presence of neck pain, if you use some caution about the vigor with which you go after them and follow the principles of good body mechanics. Use of a soft cervical collar may be protective and comfortable during such activities.

One reason many people forsake their recreational activities when they have neck pain is that they feel guilty about pursuing pleasure activities while they are avoiding responsibility at work or at home because of pain. While the commitment to become well and fully participate in life must include responsibilities, it should include fun, too.

Sometimes the fears that have built up can be dispelled first and easiest by trying some of the fun things. You should make a list of all the things you have given up because of neck pain. This should include both tasks that you feel you should do and fun things that you would like to do. Except for the things clearly out of bounds because of extreme neck stress, you should work on that list, doing each of those things. Do them in moderation, as has been discussed, but do them. Dispel the fear of trying, and get them off the list of things you can't do anymore because of neck pain. If they cause you some pain the first time you try, don't give up—try a little smaller dose the next time. Chances are that the list has been getting longer and longer up until now. Now is the time to make it start getting smaller. You can't start doing everything right now just because you want to, but what a great thing to just reverse that direction and start making the list of things you can't do shorter after all this time of having it get longer.

chapter ten
OCCUPATIONAL AND LEGAL QUESTIONS

In one way or another, neck pain frequently relates in some way to the performance of job activity. When it does, legal questions of responsibility of employer, employee, and government agencies arise.

Work injury questions may be asked to determine if the neck pain is related to an on-the-job injury. If so, are any future problems with the neck related to that injury? Can the employee return to the regular job? Is the employer obliged to take him back? Can the employee return to some work but not the old job? Is the employer obliged to provide a modified job? Does the employer have the right to dismiss an employee who says he can't do his full job, or if he demonstrates that he can't, or if his doctor says he can't? Can a doctor make an accurate prediction of what job a patient can do? Can a government agency establish accurate guidelines outlining what work a neck pain patient can do? Must an employer provide working conditions to improve the chance of function without neck pain? Does a union provide protection of the rights of spine-injured workers? Do union requirements of narrowly defined job responsibilities get in the way of compromises, which might otherwise be made between employer and employee, to provide a satisfactory work situation?

Do attorneys protect the interest of neck-injured workers

enough to justify their cost? Do attorneys suggest or encourage neck-injured people to be more disabled than they want to be and discourage them from returning to work? Do employers who are insured really want injured employees back if the insurance company will pick up the bill anyway? Do insurance companies really care if injured workers return, if costs are passed on to the insured anyway? Are insurance adjusters honest with neck-injured workers in predicting their future difficulty when making settlements or seeking releases?

Do doctors subject injured workers to more tests and more treatments because insurance companies are paying the bill? Do doctors give injured workers less time and thoroughness of examination because they assume patients are exaggerating the symptoms when they say the injury happened at work? Do employers want some neck and back patients to be off the job longer and have more trouble so the patients can get social security disability benefits, reducing the employer's obligation? Is anyone totally disabled because of neck pain? Do disability payments require total disability or disability for the customary job? Do the terms of disability policies encourage patients to exaggerate their neck trouble so that the minimum time of disability will be exceeded?

When it is considered that some disability payments are tax free, do some workers make more money by being off than by working? Do spouses and family discourage injured workers from getting well when the injured is home to help out with the kids and do housework, farming, or other nonpublic work, while collecting disability payments? Do retirement benefits and social security regulations sometimes work together to encourage people to retire early because of disability? Do co-workers pressure injured workers to remain off or to exaggerate their trouble because of their own frustrations with the job?

Do companies have the right to maintain hiring practices to exclude certain people because they might be at increased risk for neck or back pain? If disc problems are usually the result of gradual wearing out of discs over long periods of time and seldom the result of a single injury, should employers have to compensate employees for disc trouble that became symptomatic at work? If so, should that compensation just be for time off and medical expense or should it include additional compensation? If it includes additional compensation, is that compensation meant to cover the possibility of any future episodes of trouble, or is each new episode to be considered a new injury eligible for additional compensation? Are the laws and insurance regulations such that people with gradually increasing neck pain of unknown cause are strongly influenced to assign the onset of it to some incident that happened at work?

These and many other social and legal questions repeatedly arise in relation to neck and back pain. Considerable controversy exists about the answers to all of these questions. They are not given consistent answers by doctors, lawyers, insurance executives, management or labor leaders, judges, government leaders, or patients. The answers as they apply to any one patient will vary depending on who asks the question to whom and under what circumstances. The laws that govern these situations vary considerably from state to state and country to country and are subject to frequent change and variation in interpretation.

Getting some of these questions answered is a necessary part of the solution of neck pain for many people. Considering the complexity of this situation and the hopeless, powerless feeling most people have in trying to look out for themselves through all this, getting these answers as soon as practical gives people considerable advantages in resolving their problem.

WHIPLASH?

Another common legal question related to neck pain involves the concept of "whiplash." The term is derived from the idea that passengers in a vehicle that is rapidly accelerated or decelerated have their necks injured because their heads move at a different speed than their bodies, causing their necks to crack like a whip. Actually, the rapid force on the neck would be in only one direction when only one collision occurs, not forward and then backward as with a whip. Only if two collisions occurred could the forces be at all similar.

The term most commonly arises when passengers in a slow moving or stationary vehicle are injured when a more rapidly moving vehicle strikes them from behind. This results in the lower body being thrust rapidly forward while the head tends to remain at rest, putting a sudden extension strain on the neck. The idea that the head then snaps forward with enough force to do further injury is not well-reasoned under most circumstances. The injury, therefore, is usually a simple extension injury. Whether this results in fracture or dislocation, muscle and ligament injury only, or no significant injury depends upon the force of the injury, the condition of the neck prior to the injury, and some details of posture and angle of force.

To say that such an injury is or is not a "whiplash" injury really says nothing about the type, severity, or consequence of the injury. Use of the term may create the illusion that an injury, the effects of which are not well demonstrated on examination, is better understood than it actually is.

Because the term "whiplash" presents a rather dramatic image, the term has gained popularity when legal questions of the seriousness of neck injury arise. It has come into such widespread use, in fact, that the abuses associated with it are often the subject of humor.

Unfortunately, the abuse of "whiplash" to be rewarded compensatory damages out of proportion to the seriousness of the injury has resulted in those who do have serious injuries from such mechanisms being mistreated, ignored, or accused of deception.

Use of the term by doctors, lawyers, and insurance agents may also convey to the patient the idea that the injury is more serious than the actual medical findings suggest. The anxiety resulting from fears that the problem will be permanent or may get worse, along with the tension generated by legal questions of compensation and responsibility, may perpetuate any pain that would have gone away under more relaxed circumstances. If questions of fitness for work, advice from family and friends, information about the legal contingencies of the problem from lawyers, questions of prognosis, tests, and treatments by doctors are all added in, the tension generated can become enough to cause neck pain without any injury.

GETTING IT RESOLVED

Many people become preoccupied with their involvement in the legal–social–occupational aspects of their neck problem. They become so involved in this web and so obligated to spouse, attorney, co-worker, union representative, and whomever that this preoccupation would make becoming well very difficult.

Very little is gained by preoccupation with these factors and undue prolongation of their resolution. Sometimes additional financial gain or advantage in dealing with government agencies can be gained, but the gain is seldom worth the price.

There are unfair hiring practices and re-employment policies of some companies as they relate to individuals with back and neck disorders. These practices are an unfortunate but undeniable fact of life in our society that is not apt to change soon.

The best thing most injured workers can do to protect their occupational futures is to make a real effort to return to whatever work they are capable of doing as soon after the injury as they can safely do so. Prolonged and repeated absences from work make a successful occupational future less likely.

Doctor-imposed restrictions on work capacity may narrow workers' options in their jobs or in the job market. A very high percentage of workers are too stiff, too weak, too overweight, or have too little stamina to be permitted unrestricted work, yet because the question has never arisen, they do not have to deal with employers with the stigma of a medical restriction. Sometimes a necessary part of the resolution of the problem is for doctors to answer questions about restriction as best they can. Often though, the statement of a medical restriction is not really essential. If the employee learns the principles of good body mechanics and makes a full effort at rehabilitation, the need to restrict certain activities at work will be apparent and gradually diminish. Employers and co-workers who wish to encourage the rehabilitation of injured workers can help out by modifying aspects of the job and giving an extra hand during the recovery phase. These adjustments are usually far superior to some artificially determined limitation that may carry a stamp of permanence.

Whatever adjustments are made, the neck and back pain sufferer is the one who ends up with the consequences. Long after the doctors and lawyers are paid and the insurance companies and employers have discharged what is determined to be their responsibility, the patient is left with the consequences. If those consequences are loss of a good job, loss of power in the job market, and loss of the sense of accomplishment, fellowship, and other benefits that most people derive from regular work, the price has been too high for what was gained. If the adjustments lead the patient to forsake a path of wellness for one of the chronic neck pain patient with all the consequences described in the various sections of this text, the price will certainly have been exorbitant.

No one is in a position to look out for your interests like you are. If you know the full score and take an honest look at the short- and long-term consequences of the choices you must make, you have done what you can. You need to get those concerns behind you as fast as the system will allow you with the decisions you make. Whatever the financial and social consequences of your decisions, do not pay the price of good health.

chapter eleven
EXERCISE INTRODUCTION

Almost everything you hear or read about neck care advises some form of exercise. Yet some people feel that the neck pain began in the first place because of exercise, or that they have tried exercise and gotten no better or worse, or that exercise just seems impossible. To some, learning all the ways to keep from straining the neck and then being advised to exercise it seem inconsistent. But there is a great deal of misunderstanding about what is meant by exercise and how it applies to neck problems. Once understood, the importance of exercise to a healthy neck is apparent.

Some exercises can produce stresses that could cause the neck to hurt, maybe even the same stresses that led to the neck problem in the first place. The difference between accepting these stresses in the form of exercise and allowing them to occur at other times is that with exercise the stress is monitored and controlled. By slowly building up to and beyond the point where injury might have occured, you make the supporting structures ready to accept the stress without ill effect.

The need to avoid excess stress, as taught in the sections on posture and body mechanics, and the need to develop tolerance to stress, as taught in the section on exercise, are not contradictory. The two needs must be balanced and coordinated. Both techniques must be learned and applied together as is right for you at the time.

What posture and mechanical stress is acceptable and what exercise level is desirable change all the time—with proper application they change in the direction that provides better function and less pain.

There are, of course, many different types of exercise. An almost endless variation on activities can be termed exercise. Exercises may, however, be divided into a small number of groups, depending on the goal of the exercise. We will want to consider five groups: exercises done for *posture*, those done for *relaxation*, those that promote motion and *flexibility*, those that build *strength*, and those that produce *general fitness*.

Many exercise activities lead toward more than one of these goals. Each person will have different goals and will have different capabilities to use the exercises that help achieve those goals. Exercise prescriptions are, therefore, not the same for everyone. Nor will the exercise program and the goals always be the same for the same person. By understanding the goals and the principles of the exercises that lead to their achievement, you will be able to choose what will be safest, most effective, and most pleasant for you. Then, as you make progress, you will be able to adjust your exercise program to tailor it to your needs.

chapter twelve
EXERCISES FOR POSTURE

Poor posture habits may result from weak muscles, tight muscles or joints, psychological problems, habit, overweight, ignorance of good posture, and, often, a combination of these factors.

Correction of poor posture habits, regardless of their cause, can improve or prevent neck pain, back pain, and headache. The correction will be aided by direct attack on the underlying problems by strengthening weak muscles and stretching tight muscles. In this section, however, we will consider some shortcutting exercises that go directly to the posture problem.

The "scapula squeeze" is a basic neck posture exercise. The shoulder blades are central to neck posture, being between the lumbar and cervical spine. So by positioning them properly, the neck, low back, and arms fall into better position.

First "protract" the scapulae by pointing forward as far as you can with both shoulders. As you do this you can feel the scapulae glide forward across the back and side of the chest. Then pull them back. Feel them come together in the middle of the back so the skin folds in the middle. Then drop the shoulders and relax, leaving the scapulae back.

You don't want to try to keep the scapulae squeezed all the time, but you should do this exercise frequently throughout the day. Repeated movement and use of the muscles that control the scapulae keep them from knotting in spasm. The feel of having the scapulae back gives the feel of good posture. While you don't want to keep them forced back all the time, you do want them relaxed near that position most of the time.

Tucking the chin in is another exercise for posture that can and should be done repeatedly throughout the day. It can be done at the same time as the scapula squeeze. To tuck the chin in, bring the head back over the shoulders, then draw the chin in. As you draw the chin in you feel the back of the neck stretch. This stretches the muscles of the back of the neck, helping them to relax. It also brings the head back over the shoulders and chest where the muscles of the back of the neck don't have to pull so hard.

Just as you don't want to keep your scapulae squeezed all the time, you don't want to keep your chin tucked, like a military cadet, all the time. You do want to move your chin, frequently, into that posture and then relax a little, leaving it near that position, without forcing it.

The third postural exercise that should be done repeatedly through the day for the stretching effect and to make the position habitual is the "pelvic tilt." Stand slouched against a wall and reach in behind your back feeling the space between the low back and the wall. Now squeeze the buttocks together and suck the stomach in. As you do so, feel your pelvis tilt forward. Flatten your low back against the wall. This "pelvic tilt" position straightens the lumbar (low back) spine and makes a more stable, upright base for the upper spine. Notice that the lower edge of the ribs in front is further from the pelvis, leaving more room to take big, relaxed breaths.

The three posture exercises—scapula squeeze, chin in, and pelvic tilt—can be combined all at once into the overall posture exercise: "getting tall" (see Figure 10). If you do all these exercises properly, at the same time, you will actually get taller. Stand next to the wall and measure to see it for yourself.

One way to practice getting tall is to imagine that there is a wire attached to the middle of the top of your head (see Figure 4). Imagine a gentle but firm upward pull so that the weight of your head is overcome, your neck is pulled up straight and in line with your back, your pelvis swings forward and your low back

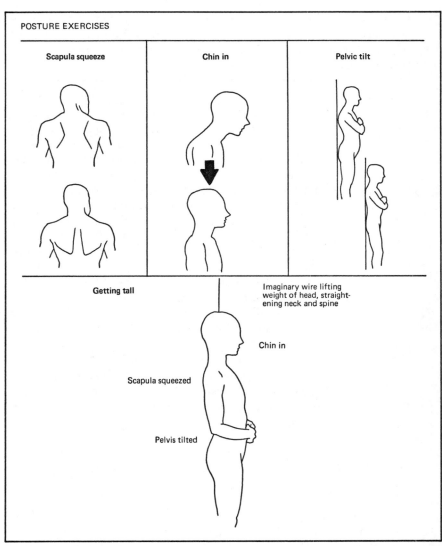

Figure 10 Posture Exercises

straightens. Once you get this help to get you tall then you can relax a little—let your jaw loosen so your teeth are not touching, let your shoulders drop down (but not forward) and breathe deeply and easily.

Another imagination trick to help with keeping the correct posture is to imagine that you have a "third eye" (see Figure 4). The "third eye" is located just below the Adam's apple in the little notch above where the collar bones come together in front. If you keep your head and shoulders up and back so the "third eye" can always see well, you will maintain good neck and shoulder posture.

Once you get the feel of these postural exercises, you will enjoy doing them repeatedly throughout the day. They are easy, low-energy activities and can be accomplished many times without exhaustion or fear of overworking the muscles. Make a habit of doing them during idle moments, in response to twinges of pain, or in preparation for any stressful activity.

chapter thirteen
RELAXATION EXERCISES

Most people feel the tensions that build up as a result of the demands and frustrations of life. Tensions aren't always felt in the same way. Sometimes they may be felt as headache, sometimes as nervousness, sometimes as fatigue. Often the result is muscle tenseness.

Muscle tenseness or muscle tension may gradually build without you being aware of its presence. By the time tension is causing pain, it may have been present a long while and may be pretty severe. Then the pain that tension causes is one more frustration leading to more tension, more pain, and on it goes.

Neck pain is a frequent component of this cycle. Sometimes tension is the most important factor in neck pain and almost always it is at least some portion of the problem. Even pains caused by such obviously explainable things as broken bones or operations are made much worse by tension.

Learning to recognize and control some of the frustrations that lead to tensions is one means of interrupting the tension–pain–tension cycle. That approach is discussed in the section on psychological factors.

Another approach is to recognize the muscle tension when it starts to build and to learn to apply techniques to relax the muscles before the tension begins to make the pain worse.

Some people object to calling relaxation techniques "exercise." They fear that just the mention of exercise may cause tension and make relaxation hard. One of the things you want, however, is to dispel any notions you have of exercise being unpleasant. Different forms of exercise produce feelings of well-being and relaxation in different ways and at different times. Fitness and strengthening exercises, done properly, leave you with those feelings afterward. Relaxation exercises are meant to help you achieve those feelings directly during the exercise period, ideally with a carry-over effect into the rest of the day.

Like the posture exercises, relaxation exercises can be done as often as you wish without fear of overdoing. They should be done at times when you feel the tension building, at times and in situations that you have observed tension building, and when you want to be fully relaxed, such as before beginning stretching and strengthening exercises.

Performing a little experiment to demonstrate the effects of tension is helpful. Stand with your back flat against the wall, then move your feet out about one step, bending the knees, and lowering your buttocks a little more than halfway down to sitting posture. See how long you can stay there. The answer will depend on your state of conditioning, how far you bend your knees, and your pain tolerance, but it won't be long. The pain you feel in the big muscles in the front of your thighs is the result of sustained muscle tension. It's not hard to understand how the muscles of the jaw, neck, and shoulders cause pain if, for whatever reason, they are maintained in a tense state for long.

Many different techniques or exercises are designed to achieve relaxation. Variations on commonly used ones are presented here as examples. Most people can effectively employ these techniques on their own. The use of tapes, equipment such as biofeedback devices, and professional guidance (as from a psychologist, psychiatrist, or physical therapist) can increase the proficiency with which these methods are used and are recommended for those who cannot achieve the desired result on their own.

The first relaxation exercise to be described, the contrast-relaxation exercise, is not only an effective tool to achieve relaxation, but also another demonstration of the feel of muscle tension.

CONTRAST-RELAXATION EXERCISES

Obtain a quiet room away from phone, television, radio, or other distractions. A tape to guide you through the exercise or soft instrumental music may be played, but otherwise silence is best. Dim the lights, loosen tight clothing, and remove tight or heavy jewelry. Lie in the rest position on a rug or exercise mat.

Take three deep, easy breaths. You are going to alternately tighten and relax various muscles. By doing so, you will learn the feeling of tension and the feeling of relaxation. Tighten muscles gradually at first. Do not make them hurt. Continue to breathe deeply and easily throughout the exercise.

Tighten the right hand into a fist. Hold for five seconds, thinking "my hand is tense." Then let go and let the fingers fall loose and limp. Think "my fingers are warm and relaxed." Do this three times, then repeat with the left hand three times.

Now raise the right arm up, clench the fist, bend the elbow by forcing the fist to the shoulder, and tighten all the shoulder and neck muscles. Hold five seconds, thinking "my arm is tense." Then let the arm flop down. Think "my arm is heavy, warm, and relaxed." After three times with the right arm, do the same three times with the left arm.

Move the ankles, heels, and knees together so they touch one another. Now squeeze them as tightly together as you can. Start with the ankles, then, keeping the ankles tight, force the knees tightly together. Keep knees and ankles tightly squeezed together, then tighten the buttock muscles together. Hold everything tight for five seconds, thinking "my legs are tense." Then suddenly relax all the muscles. Feel the heaviness of the legs and of your hips against the floor. Think "my legs are heavy, warm, and relaxed."

Now shrug your shoulders up to your ears. Press your shoulder blades and upper back down, hard against the floor. Think "my back is tense." Hold five seconds. Then let it all go and feel your back and shoulders sink. Think "my back is heavy, warm, and relaxed."

Push the back of your head down tightly against the floor. Tense the neck muscles in front and back, clenching the teeth. Think "my neck is tense." Now relax. Feel your head heavy against the floor. Feel the heaviness of your jaw as it drops open and your teeth separate. Tell yourself "my head is heavy, warm, and relaxed."

Pucker up your lips very tightly and hold three seconds, then relax and let the lips go slack. Then, pull the mouth into a deep frown. Hold three seconds feeling the tension, then let go. Smile broadly three seconds, then let go. Wrinkle up the nose three seconds, then let it relax. Raise the eyebrows and tense the wrinkles in the forehead three seconds—then let them go and let the forehead smooth. Squint the eyes tightly shut. Hold them three seconds, then relax, letting the lids droop almost closed. Now tense all the face muscles together and hold five seconds. Then relax. Feel your forehead go smooth and all tension leave your face. Feel your teeth separate and your tongue feel heavy in the floor of your mouth. Repeat this three times.

Now lie quietly, limp and free. Feel the heaviness of your arms, legs, and head, the smoothness of your face. Breathe easily and deeply, saying to yourself with each breath, "relax." Learn this feeling of being relaxed so you can recall it anytime during your day.

This series of exercises and others using the same principles are called "contrast-relaxation exercises." By consciously tensing the muscles so you can really feel them tense, you can become aware of that tense feeling and then can contrast that with the relaxation that follows. The same principle can be used to obtain relaxation in various situations throughout the day without having to interrupt for an exercise session.

MEDITATION

Meditation is often associated with mystical, spiritual, or exotic practices. Those associations may be so, but not necessarily. Unless combined with spiritual or mystical elements, meditation is a simple, healthful practice which is unusual only in its contrast to the pace of the rest of contemporary society.

The purpose of meditation is to calm the mind by limiting attention to a single focus. This may involve chanting a word or focusing on a spiritual image, but when meditating for practical, healthful purposes you usually focus on the breath. All of the mind's usual chatter and static of worries, plans, and fantasies are regarded as intrusions on the process of concentrating on this one subject—the breath. Any other neutral, always available subject or image can be chosen if you have any reason to prefer it to the breath.

Meditation is a skill to be learned and practiced. Devotion of time and effort are required. Until mastered, meditation should be practiced at least daily, preferably at the same time and in the same place. Allow 20 minutes. Make every effort to secure freedom from interruptions and intruding noises. Use a timer so you know when the time is up without having to periodically check.

Begin with an alert mind. Don't practice meditation at a time when you are usually sleepy. You can meditate recumbent or seated in the classic "lotus" position, but for most novices meditation is best done seated in a straight chair with a comfortably padded but hard seat.

Sit so the front edge of the chair strikes you at midthigh. The height of the chair should be such that the knees are at about hip height. Have both feet flat on the floor so the angle between the lower legs and thighs is a little more than 90 degrees. Let the arms hang limp at the side and hold the lower back comfortably straight. Rock back and forth a little until you find a neutral, balanced position. Next, allow your head to roll about over your shoulders a little until it, too, finds a neutral position over the shoulders. Now lift your hands and allow them to flop across your inner thighs so the weight of your forearms comes to rest on your thighs.

This neutral, balanced sitting posture can be used as a starting point for contrast-relaxation exercises, deep relaxation, or meditation.

Close your eyes and pay attention to your breathing. Follow each breath all the way in and all the way out. Think only of the breathing. If any other thought comes to mind, allow it to pass right on through. Every other thought should only be a reminder to return your concentration to the breathing.

You may wish to count the breaths. Count up to 10 and then start over. You may want to incorporate some word or image into the counting. Use of such a "mantra" may allow you to recall this word in times of stress and, with it, recall some of the feelings of serenity you experience while meditating.

You may also use the image of some surrounding color—usually a restful color such as blue or green—a technique sometimes called "chromotherapy." You may imagine the pain as a harsh color and then think of drops falling into it, fading it, then converting it to a restful color.

Whether you count, use a word or phrase in rhythm, or use some visual image with the breathing, such techniques should only compliment your attention to the breathing. No thoughts of productivity or obligation, no worries, no longings or regrets are to intrude on this concentration on the breathing. Every such thought reminds you to think only of the breathing and then passes right on by.

When you have completed your meditation time, open your eyes. Look at and sense your body. Note how relaxed you are. Stretch and arise alert and relaxed.

Those who meditate regularly do so because they feel less stress and are able to maintain tension-free alertness more successfully when they do so. The benefits are more apparent after weeks of practice. Concentrating and achieving full benefit from the technique are often difficult at first. Once mastered, however, the technique may be recalled, like typing or riding a bicycle, with much greater ease than that with which it was first learned.

DEEP RELAXATION

Another deep relaxation technique involves some elements of both the contrast-relaxation and meditation exercises. This technique is more complex, so having an assistant read the instructions or using a tape until the technique is mastered is best. This technique may be done in various positions. The instructions vary depending on the position. To provide something different from the back-lying and the sitting position, the following instruction for this type of exercise is given for lying on the right side of a bed. The floor or an exercise mat can be used as an alternate surface.

You should be in a quiet, dimly lit room. All outside thoughts and worries should pass right through without you thinking about them. Assure that you will not be interrupted.

Lie on your right side with a small, soft pillow under the right side of the head. Both legs are bent at the knee, and the left leg is pulled up higher toward the chest and rests on a pillow in front of the right leg. The right arm is behind the back with the elbow bent comfortably, the back of the hand against the bed and the fingers open. The left arm is in front with the hand palm down at face level.

Feel the heaviness of your body against the bed. Feel that heaviness sink your body down into the bed. Don't be afraid. Let it go heavier and heavier, deeper and deeper. Don't force it, just let it happen. Feel your weight pulled down. Feel your eyes loose and heavy. Your forehead is smooth and wide. Your lips are limp. Your teeth are apart. Push your tongue hard against the roof of your mouth, harder and harder. Feel it tense your facial muscles, even down into your neck and chest. Now let your tongue fall, heavy and limp, down against the teeth on the right side of the mouth. Feel how heavy your tongue is. Feel how relaxed your face and head are.

You let yourself be more relaxed than before. You are heavier, sinking deeper. Now feel where the right foot touches the bed. Feel the contact. Feel the heaviness. Feel the pull, the binding between the foot and the bed. Feel the foot sink into the bed, become part of it. Now feel the right knee and everywhere that touches between the foot and the knee. Feel the leg and floor pull together. Feel the leg flow into the bed and become part of it. Now feel the right hip. Feel the heaviness of the pelvis pushing down, and the hip flowing into and sinking into the bed. Feel the upper leg. Feel where the foot touches the bed. Feel it flow into the bed, sinking down and becoming part of it. Feel the heaviness all along the left leg as it flows into the pillow. Everywhere the leg touches it sinks down in. Feel the heaviness of the left hip and the thigh as it sinks down. As the hip and thigh become more limp, heavier, they push the right side further down, making it heavier and sinking it deeper into the bed.

Now feel all along the side and the chest. Feel the heaviness, feel the pull down, down into the bed. Feel the muscles let go under the collar bone. The left side of the chest is loose and heavy and falls down against the right chest, which is sinking heavier into the bed. Feel the right shoulder being pulled down where it touches—sinking, binding, becoming part of the bed. Feel the same heaviness all along the right arm where it lies against the bed. The arm is heavy, pulled down into the bed. Feel the back of the hand heavy, sinking down and down, flowing into the bed where it touches. Feel the fingers open and loose. Feel the blood flow through the finger tips, making them warm and relaxed. The left shoulder is heavy, loose, sinking down, pushing the right shoulder down deeper. The left arm, all along where it touches the bed, becomes heavier and heavier. The arm is sinking in. The left hand is heavy, the palm sinking in, becoming part of the bed. The finger tips are warm where they touch. The blood flowing in them warms them and the warmness flows into the bed.

Your head is very heavy, sinking down, down into the pillow. It is pulled down, flowing into the pillow. You let it go. You feel your head let go under your ears, behind the base of your skull. You are not afraid. You allow yourself to sink deeper. Your cheeks and lips sag. Your tongue is heavy, drooping against the side of your teeth. Your eyelids are heavy. Your forehead is smooth. You sink deeper and deeper. You are not afraid. You are completely relaxed. Remain that way for a moment then stretch and arise, refreshed and relaxed.

KEEP TENSION IN BALANCE

Few people can spend their lives meditating and devoting full attention to relaxation. Everyone, though, needs some break from the tensions that develop from their lives. Many of the things that bring on the tensions are things that are also pleasurable and profitable—spouses, kids, jobs. So tension is not always avoidable. By learning these relaxation techniques, you will have a way to give your muscles a break from the tension.

chapter fourteen
EXERCISES FOR FLEXIBILITY

Stiffness may result from limited joint motion, limited ability of the muscles and tendons to stretch, or both. Lack of exercise and tension are the major culprits in development of stiffness.

Stretching beyond the limit of easy motion usually involves some discomfort. Even the perfectly healthy people who have never had anything wrong with neck muscles or joints have pain when stressed beyond what they are accustomed to. Any such healthy person trying to do "the splits" for the first time would certainly experience pain, and were the splits accomplished, would probably experience serious injury. Very few people are born able to do the splits. Most of those who can became able to do so by patient, careful, repeated effort.

The same patient, careful, repeated effort that enables people to learn to move joints and muscles beyond what is "normal" can bring back lost normal motion.

Stiff muscles and joints hurt when stretched even within a usual or "normal" range. That is one good reason to exercise—to try to gain flexibility and eliminate stiffness. There is more reason than that, however.

Loss of normal motion prevents normal posture. Muscles and joints work together in ways so that loss of normal motion in one muscle may result in loss of some motion in the joint it crosses.

This, in turn, causes other joints to position themselves abnormally to compensate. If the lower back is stiff, for example, the neck is strained to maintain upper body position without the help it usually gets from shifts of position made in the lower spine.

WORDS OF CAUTION AND PATIENCE

Moving joints of the neck beyond the range to which they are accustomed can be hazardous in unusual situations. Those who are known to have a lot of bone spurs, arthritis, or spondylosis—especially elderly people or those troubled by dizziness related to neck position—should never forcefully bend the head and neck backward beyond what is customary. Those with arm pain, numbness, and/or weakness in the lower arm and hand should not undergo sudden, forceful rotations of the head.

These precautions are given to emphasize the need to proceed carefully in certain unusual situations. Actually, sudden forceful movements are not the keys to increased flexibility regardless of the underlying problem. Patient repetition is the key.

Motion is lost because of prolonged tension, underexercise, poor posture, and, in some instances, disorders of the underlying anatomy. These changes almost always occur slowly. Even if the symptoms begin abruptly, the changes that cause persisting stiffness occur slowly over a long time. You cannot reverse those changes rapidly. Regaining motion takes time and a lot of patience and persistence.

Exercises to gain motion (flexibility exercises) should be done as a concentrated effort at least twice a day. Even then, however, people have a great tendency to stiffen up in between exercise sessions. At least some brief modification of the exercises should be done every waking hour until motion is regained. You can learn to make exercises a habit for idle moments and to do them without major interruption of your daily activities.

Flexibility exercises, when done as a concentrated effort to push beyond the easy range of motion, should not be done until the body area is "warmed up." If they are done early in the morning, they should follow several minutes of warm-up activity in which the muscles are used within their comfortable range or following a general fitness exercise. When done later in an active day, exercises require less warm-up, but motion should not be forced into a stiff muscle or joint as an initial exercise.

Exercise sessions that attempt to stretch more motion into stiff, sore muscles may be more effective if heat is applied first, using the techniques described in the chapter on first aid. Warm clothing also helps. After a long session of stretching exercises, you may find it helpful to put an ice pack on the areas that have been sore.

ACTIVE AND PASSIVE EXERCISES

Several types of exercises may help with flexibility. "Passive exercises" are those that are done by someone else to you with no effort on your part except to relax. Passive exercise has the disadvantage of requiring the presence of someone else. That person must be helpful, but gentle, and must understand that sudden jerking, forceful motions are not helpful and could be harmful.

Exercises done purely on your own are called "active exercises." Pure active exercise involves only the use of your own muscles to exert the force.

Many exercises combine active and passive elements. Using gravity props such as a desk or edge of a bed to exert more force than you are exerting with your muscles is a common form of partially active, partially passive exercise. This is a form of "active assisted exercise."

When help is available, another form of "active assisted exercise" may be done. The basic effort comes from active muscle push, but a little extra push, or assist in holding what has been gained, is added by an assistant.

The specific exercises recommended to accomplish increased motion in the various planes of the various joints depend upon the beginning capabilities of the person. While almost everyone can do the posture exercises previously described, the flexibility and strengthening exercises need to be more individually tailored.

NECK MOVEMENTS

The neck moves forward into "flexion," and backward into "extension." The movements occur in segments at each level that the vertebrae join together. The higher segments bend the head forward by tucking the chin in, and the lower segments bend it by nodding the head forward on the chest. More total flexion is possible if the chin is tucked in first and the head then nodded.

The head moves sideways into "lateral tilt" by leaning the head so that the ear touches the shoulder. Neck motion also occurs in "rotation" by turning the chin to touch the shoulder. Rotation naturally involves some lateral bending (toward the opposite shoulder) at the same time.

The neck can also be made to seem to shift directly forward and backward and side to side without appreciable tilting. Such movement is common to many dance forms. Such "carrying movements" or "translational shifts" are really well-controlled combinations of the other movements. Practicing them is good exercise for movement and control of the neck.

Once the various movements of the neck are known, the exercises to maintain or increase the range of these movements are fairly obvious. The variations depend upon body position and whether any assistive force is applied.

Active Exercises for Neck Flexion and Extension

In trying to gain as much flexion and extension as possible, you may find isolating the effort on various segments by varying the position of the chin helpful. Tucking the chin, and, conversely, tucking the occiput (base of the skull) in above the shoulder blades forces motion into the upper neck. Reaching as far down the breast bone (sternum) as possible with the chin, and as far down the back between the shoulder blades (scapulae) as possible puts stretch on the lower neck.

Gravity against the weight of the head supplies some assistive force, so if you must begin very gently, you may do best to begin lying down so only the active force of your own muscles is applied (see Figure 11).

If, on the other hand, you don't need to be gentle and you need more force to improve the motion, you can clasp your hands in front of the forehead or behind the head and add the force of arm weight to the effort.

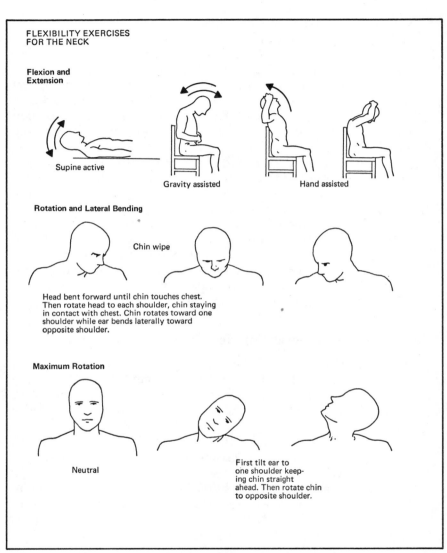

Figure 11 Flexibility Exercises for the Neck

Active Exercises for Neck Rotation and Lateral Bending

The combination of bending the head to the side and rotating the neck can be practiced using the "chin wipe" exercise (see Figure 11). Imagine something is on the underside of your chin and try to wipe it off by rubbing it across your chest from one shoulder to the other.

This simple chin wipe exercise, along with seated flexion and extension of the head, can be done in a few seconds, inconspicuously and without special preparation. Repeating this every waking hour maintains the progress toward flexibility that is made with the more prolonged and vigorous exercises.

A more forceful active exercise to improve rotation is done by first tilting the ear to the shoulder with the chin comfortably up and straight ahead. When maximum lateral bending brings the ear as close as possible to the shoulder, then turn the chin toward the opposite shoulder (see Figure 11). Doing the exercise in this sequence positions the neck for the greatest potential rotation.

To gain maximum lateral bending, rotate the chin fully to the opposite shoulder, then tilt the ear toward the near shoulder.

Passive Flexibility Exercises

Discussion of passive neck motion exercise can be found in the chapter on first aid. Some discussion is repeated here because passive exercises can help regain flexibility. The same techniques and precautions apply. Many people with neck pain and stiffness have more passive motion without pain than they are able to perform by active techniques.

Passive motion exercises are done lying down or in a reclining position, with the helper standing near the head.

Movement is preceded by massaging the muscles of the shoulders, base of the head, and back and sides of the neck. Then a gentle stretching pull is applied from the back of the neck as if to stretch the neck out longer. Alternate pulling for 10 seconds with relaxation. Then begin to gently tilt, rotate, flex, and extend the head with the pull.

Just as with active movements, the level of mobilization can be varied by varying the position of the chin.

More total rotation can be achieved by tilting the head maximally to the opposite side first. More total flexion can be achieved by tucking the chin in first.

Extremes of extension should be avoided. Anything painful should be avoided. Sudden jerking and excessive force should not be used.

You generally do best to develop increased motion first in directions in which you have no discomfort. Thus, if it hurts to rotate to the left, try to obtain full rotation to the right before trying to increase the tolerance to left rotation.

Passive motion, like long sessions of active motion efforts, can be used on a once or twice a day basis to try to increase motion. Maintenance of those gains is provided by hourly active exercise sessions of a few seconds duration.

EXERCISES FOR THE SHOULDER

Loss of shoulder motion often accompanies neck pain. The neck problem may cause the shoulder problem or vice versa, or the two may be present at the same time, but not related by any known cause. The association is so common that shoulder movement needs to be understood by all people with neck pain, and shoulder flexibility exercises should be done by those with shoulder pain and those who have any hint of loss of any of the shoulder movements.

The shoulder moves forward and back into "flexion" and "extension." It moves across and out to the side of the body into "adduction" and "abduction." The shoulder rotates across the body into "internal rotation" as though to put the hand behind the back, and outward into "external rotation" in the manner of a hitchhiker.

These movements can be combined to produce a rolling motion similar to bending forward making circles with the hand while the arm is down straight. This motion is called "circumduction." Another complex combination of these movements results in the ability to reach for the ceiling, or "overhead extension." Those with shoulder pain need to take the shoulder through the full range of all of these movements at least twice daily. Preventing loss of shoulder motion is much easier than trying to regain it once it is lost.

If shoulder motion has already been lost, you may need to have someone help provide passive motion. Several devices (see Figure 12) may be helpful.

Gravity and the pendulum effect may be used to supplement muscle effort by doing "circumduction exercises." The pendulum effect can be increased in flexion and extension by holding a weight such as a vegetable can in the hand.

If you "climb up a wall" with the fingers, you can hold each step of progress while preparing to take the next step. A simple pulley, a cane or broomstick, and a towel can all be used in various ways to allow the good arm to assist the effort of the bad arm to regain full shoulder motion (see Figure 12).

BACK FLEXIBILITY EXERCISES

Neck pain and back pain are frequently present at the same time or at different times in the same person. Stiffness in the lower back may result in increased tension stress on the neck. Keeping the back flexible should be part of the exercise program for all people with neck pain. Those who have had back pain may need to give special emphasis to back flexibility exercises.

From a supine (back lying) position, pull one knee upward to the chest. You should hold under the thigh just above the knee so the pull is concentrated on the hip. You will feel the pull on the muscles of the back of the hip on the lifted side. After you exceed the range of easy hip flexion on that side, you will feel the pelvis start to rotate up with the leg. You will feel the tightness as it starts to draw the front of the opposite, straight leg up. This "supine, single knee-chest lift" is a stretching exercise for tightness in the back (extensors) of the active hip and tightness in the front (flexors) of the opposite hip. Switching to the other leg completes the flexion and extension exercise of both hips.

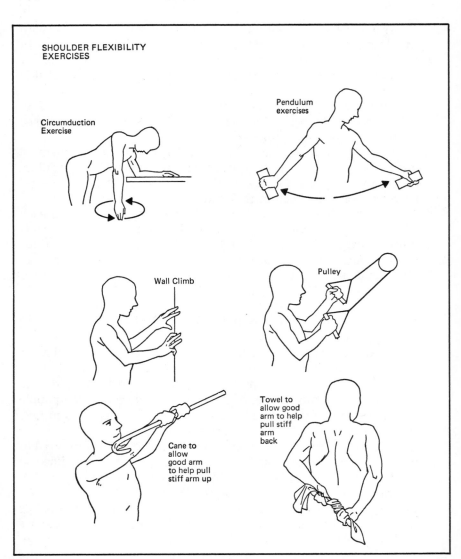

Figure 12 Shoulder Flexibility Exercises

116

If you grasp behind your knee and pull your shoulders up a little while doing the supine, single knee-chest lift, you will feel a gentle arching stretch of the lower back.

By pulling both knees up at the same time—a "supine, double knee-chest lift"—you no longer hold the pelvis down. As the limit of easy hip flexion and pelvic rotation is exceeded, the lower back is pulled into more flexion. This is a gentler and more controlled flexion exercise for the low back than is a standing toe touch. After pulling both knees to the chest, stretch them back out and down one at a time.

A slightly more demanding low back flexion and extension exercise that can be done by those who can do supine double knee-chest lifts well, but are not ready for toe touches, is the "cat back" exercise. Begin on the hands and knees. Let the back sag into lordosis as much as it comfortably will, then reverse the position of the low back by making an arched "cat back." Move the hands toward and away from the knees to shift positions. Don't try to make sudden switches from one position to the other. As with all exercises, it is best to do this in a slow, stretching, nonballistic way with easy, relaxed breathing throughout.

The same motion as the cat back and the double knee-chest lifts can be duplicated from a side-lying position. They can also be done from the seated position in a straight chair.

JAW MOTION EXERCISE

Tension and stiffness of neck muscles are often associated with tight, stiff facial muscles. Setting the jaw and clenching the teeth are tight muscle activities. Simply opening the mouth as wide as possible stretches tight jaw muscles. You should open your mouth as wide as you can several times each day. You may be surprised at how stiff the jaw muscles and the skin of the face feel when you begin doing this and how much relaxation you may feel in your neck muscles after these simple jaw stretches.

chapter fifteen
EXERCISES FOR STRENGTHENING

Making muscles stronger makes them more resistant to injury from sudden stresses. Strong muscles are more able to protect the underlying bones and ligaments from injury. Increased strength means better tone and improved ability to maintain current posture.

NECK MUSCLE STRENGTHENING

The muscles that move across the neck to control head and neck positions can be safely strengthened by contracting them against resistance supplied by the hand (see Figure 13). This "isometric" (meaning muscle contraction without movement) form of neck exercise is safe because it does not involve equipment, will not result in excessive stress in extreme positions, and allows immediate release of the resistance.

The exercises may be done seated, standing, or reclining. They may be more effective done reclining so that other muscles are relaxed and full attention can be placed upon the neck.

The muscles that flex the neck foward are resisted by placing the hands on the forehead. Force the head forward and chin down. Pull as hard as you can with the neck muscles while supplying

118

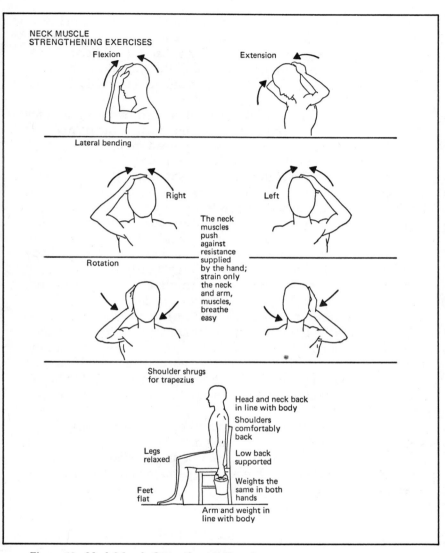

Figure 13   Neck Muscle Strengthening Exercises

119

enough resistance with your hands so that the chin does not move.

To strengthen the muscles that extend the neck backward, clasp the hands, placing the palms on the back of the head. Try to force the head backward and the base of the skull down between the shoulder blades. Apply enough hand resistance so that the head is held still.

Lateral bending muscles are strengthened by trying to force the ear directly over to the shoulder while holding the palm of the hand against the temple to prevent any head motion.

Apply the palm along the side of the jaw to supply resistance against rotation of the chin toward the shoulder.

These six isometric exercises—flexion, extension, right and left lateral bending, and right and left rotation—provide means to gain all the neck muscle strength needed for ordinary activities. Football players, wrestlers, and others who subject themselves to danger from violent injuries to the head and neck need to use body weight or exercise devices to provide extraordinary strength to neck muscles. For most people, the strength supplied by isometrics is quite adequate if the exercises are done regularly.

The contractions should be held at first for a slow count to three. As strength improves and technique is mastered, the count can be lengthened to five or more. Even while maintaining maximum effort with the muscles, normal relaxed breathing should continue. Tightening the abdomen and holding the breath while doing these contractions does not help and, for some people, may be dangerous.

The number of repetitions can be increased slowly. Begin with three and slowly work up to ten.

Once strength is gained, it can be maintained by doing the exercises every other day. Frequent repetition is not necessary for strengthening like it is for flexibility.

SHOULDER STRENGTHENING

The muscles that provide shoulder strength, particularly those around the scapula, also support the posture and movements of the neck.

The trapezius (or "trap") is the large muscle that crosses at an angle from the neck to the upper portion of the shoulder blade. If you bend your elbow, reach your hand directly back until the back of your thumb is resting on the mid-collar bone, and then squeeze down with your fingers, you will squeeze the trapezius. From the position and size of this muscle, seeing its importance in maintaining neck posture is easy.

The motion of "shrugging" the shoulders puts the trapezius muscles to work. Shoulder shrugging against resistance will strengthen them (see Figure 13). Sit with the feet flat and the back supported. Hold weights in a bucket or purse in each hand. Draw the head back over the shoulders. Pull the shoulders back into a neutral position. The scapulae do not need to be squeezed together but neither should they roll forward so the arms are out in front of the body. The weights are lifted by shrugging the shoulders. The lift is done with the elbows kept straight and with the line of the arms along the side of the chest and abdomen. Hold the position to a count of five and relax.

As with all exercises, begin with less weight and fewer repetitions than you know you can do. Once you learn the technique and have a few days to see that you will not have painful aftereffects, slowly add to the weights and number of lifts. Increase only once each week. Do the exercises every other day. A general guide to the amount of weights is that if you cannot comfortably do five repetitions you are using too much weight. If you can easily do 15, it is time to add.

Shoulder Retractions

The other major muscle group that is underexercised, but consistently overworked by postural stress, is the group that retracts the scapulae (squeezes the shoulder blades together). These muscles pass from the mid-spine to the inside edge of the scapulae. The bulk of them are called "rhomboids" though some other muscles contribute to the same action.

Repeated use of these muscles as a postural exercise has previously been emphasized. The same motion of the "scapula squeeze," when done against resistance, will strengthen these muscles.

The scapula takes a fairly wide arc in its motion across the back of the chest, so you do best to exercise the muscles in different shoulder positions (see Figure 14).

To strengthen the shoulder retractors with the arms forward, you may use a towel or anything which can be firmly grasped with both hands. Simple rubber or spring devices that provide resistance against stretching are best. Hold the object out in front of the chest and supply maximum resistance in the same way described above. Keep the neck back over the shoulders and the back in normal alignment. Don't hold the breath, strain through the abdomen, or sway the back.

The same effort needs to be applied with the shoulders already back. Lie on the back with the shoulders and elbows at right angles, in the "surrender" posture (see Figure 14). Push down against the floor with the back of your elbows, trying to pinch the shoulder blades together. Bring the chest up but don't arch your back excessively. The force comes through the arms to the elbows and should be felt where the elbows contact the floor, not at the back of the head and pelvis.

LOWER BACK MUSCLE STRENGTHENING

The lower back obtains primary muscular support from groups of muscles that connect the spine to the ribs and the pelvis.

The muscles of the abdomen are large muscles that have the potential for lending considerable support to the low back. When you hold the abdominal contents firmly, they exert a hydrostatic pressure over the whole front of the spine. When you connect the ribs in front to the front of the pelvis, they help prevent the low back from sagging into lordosis.

Unfortunately, several things may weaken abdominal muscles, depriving them of their ability to support the spine. Pregnancy, abdominal surgery, and overweight are common causes of abdominal muscle weakness. Often, simply not adequately exercising the abdominal muscles for long periods of time may lead to the trouble. Combinations of these factors are responsible for a lot of back pain. The resulting changes in posture and activity may also lead to neck pain.

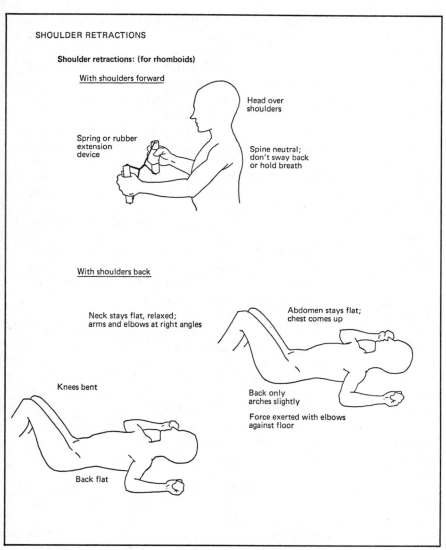

SHOULDER RETRACTIONS

Shoulder retractions: (for rhomboids)

With shoulders forward

Head over
shoulders

Spring or rubber
extension
device

Spine neutral;
don't sway back
or hold breath

With shoulders back

Neck stays flat, relaxed;
arms and elbows at right angles

Abdomen stays flat;
chest comes up

Knees bent

Back only
arches slightly

Force exerted with elbows
against floor

Back flat

Figure 14 Shoulder Retraction

Abdominal muscles stretched out by pregnancies or by too much abdominal fat lose their tone. Regaining the strength and tone needed requires a lot of effort over a long time. Sometimes the exercises needed to build back the abdominal muscles may cause some pain, but the alternative of letting the muscles get weaker and weaker and letting the abdomen protrude and allowing the back to sag can only lead to greater trouble.

The sit-up is the best exercise to strengthen abdominal muscles. Full back flexion against a tight abdomen is too much back stress for beginners and for those in pain. The straining and jerking that may accompany a full sit-up done by a beginner may be too much strain on the neck and shoulders. The benefits can be achieved without coming all the way up.

Lie on the back with knees bent and feet flat on the floor. Arms should lie comfortably along the side. Breathing is relaxed and normal. Pull smoothly up until the head and shoulders are off the surface. Feel the strain in the abdominal muscles. Hold the position, breathing normally for a second or two at first. Gradually increase the duration the position is held and the number of repetitions done.

The abdominal muscles are further strengthened through their full range with less stress to the back and neck by adding uncurls to the sit-up exercise. Do this by starting in a sitting up position, knees bent, feet flat, and arms relaxed. Lean back, holding the trunk and legs in position with the abdominal muscles. Then pull forward to sit upright. Keep feet flat and don't jerk.

When you divide the sit-up into the partial sit-up and the uncurls, the abdominal muscles can be worked through a full sit-up range without you having to bring the back and neck through a full arc.

The muscles that support the back side of the spine are called the back extensors. The exercises to strengthen them are called extension exercises. These are the muscles that are most apt to be sore in people with back pain, so exercises to strengthen them must be approached cautiously. Though a great deal of lower back support comes from the abdominal muscles, the extensor muscles are important, too, and need strengthening.

Extension exercises are done "prone" (face down). Both arms

are overhead in a relaxed "hands up" position. First bring one arm up off the floor and hold it for a second or two and then bring it down. Do the same with one leg, then the other arm, and then the other leg. Gradually add on seconds that each position is held and the number of repetitions. Progress slowly.

After gaining strength and confidence with one limb at a time, begin to lift one arm and the opposite leg together. Later, begin with both arms together and both legs together. Progress to three limbs at once and, finally, to lifting both arms and both legs at the same time.

As with all exercises, these progressions must be taken slowly. Many people have increased pain when doing sit-ups or extension exercises. The reason is that almost always the attempts at progress are too rapid. Adding on more repetitions or more difficult exercises should be done in small amounts and at weekly, not daily, intervals.

SWIMMING POOL EXERCISES

Many exercises can be done efficiently and, for some people, more pleasantly, in water. Those with regular access to a pool may use it for general fitness exercises and also for some strengthening and flexibility exercises.

While not a competitive swim stroke, the elementary back stroke provides good shoulder and upper back strengthening exercise. The arms are pulled through the water to shoulder level and then back to the sides, thereby working the muscles that support the scapulae and upper arms. The neck is maintained in a slightly flexed, neutral position, putting minimal postural stress on the upper spine.

Either a frog style or a flutter kick can be used. The frog style kick allows the lower back to stay fairly flat. This is the swimming stroke that can be done with least stress to the bones and joints of the spine.

Regulation overhead back stroke is also a good shoulder strengthening exercise. This stroke produces more extension and twisting stress to the neck than elementary back stroke, so it must be approached a bit more cautiously.

The breast stroke is an excellent scapulae-retraction strengthening exercise. For those who must avoid neck extension stress, however, the head position for breathing during the breast stroke is too stressful.

Free style swimming is good for shoulder strengthening and a good method of general fitness training. The repeated twisting of the neck for breathing may be trouble for those not yet ready for that much rotational stress to the neck.

Both free style and breast stroking may be done successfully with much less stress by using a snorkel so the head can stay beneath the water, in a near neutral position, throughout the exercise period.

As with all exercises, no one number of repetitions or duration of effort for pool exercises is correct. Begin easily and slowly, and progress as you gain strength.

BUILD SLOWLY

Remember that muscle strength building takes time. The same stresses that put tough callouses on the palms by repeated, gradual, increasing effort cause painful blisters if done too rapidly. The commitment to strength and fitness is a lifetime one. There is nothing to be gained by trying to hurry the progress beyond that for which you are prepared.

chapter sixteen
EXERCISES FOR GENERAL FITNESS

Some people seem to be able to work and live under great stress without showing the effects of tension. Some people seem to endure injuries and illnesses that must be very painful without letting pain interfere with their function and enjoyment of life. In some cases, these people are just born with high tolerance to stress and pain. Others seem to develop these abilities.

One of the characteristics of a large percentage of these people is exceptional physical fitness. Witness the pain and discomfort endured by soldiers in battle, football players, boxers, and marathon runners. They may be able to withstand injury at the moment and go on because they are "psyched up" or their "adrenalin is up," but they also seem to suffer less afterward than unfit people with similar injuries. Studies of workmen on fitness programs compared to workmen who are not so fit show that those who are fit miss far less work from comparable injuries.

Not only do those who are exceptionally well fit seem to be able to withstand physical injury better, but they tolerate stress and frustration better, have less trouble with feelings of depression, and require less sleep.

All of the reasons for these advantages of fitness are not known. One explanation is that the physical stress of regular exercise produces brain hormones that act to decrease feelings of pain.

The psychological benefits of feeling strong and capable of controlling one's body also must play some part.

It has only been in the relatively recent history of humanity that most of us, most of the time, are safe from attack. People's need to defend themselves was well served by body reflexes and reactions that prepared us for "fight or flight." These same physical mechanisms are still in our bodies and they still exert their effects when we are stressed. Only, now, the stresses are different and the solutions, when there are some, don't come from physical flight or fight. If we don't have some physical outlet to allow our body mechanisms to work the way they were made to, we don't have good health.

The sort of fitness that helps with stress and pain tolerance and decreases depression is gained by the same sort of exercise that leads to cardiorespiratory (heart and lung) fitness. These exercises improve lung function, decrease high blood pressure, and decrease the risk of death from heart attack.

Exercises to gain these advantages require at least 30 minutes at least every other day. They should be painless, though slightly stressful. The idea is to work up to and sustain an exercise program that will allow continuous, mildly stressful exercise for 30 minutes or more at a time. This is a lifetime commitment, so you would be foolish to rush into an exercise program too fast and make it unpleasant or risk injury.

The chosen exercise must be something easily controlled and rhythmic. It should be something easily accessible on a year-round, regular basis. The exercise should be easily measurable so that the amount of stress may be gradually increased. It must be something that can be continued for the entire exercise session without rest or need for sudden bursts of extra effort.

The fitness activities that qualify are jogging, swimming, bicycling, aerobic dancing, rowing, and cross country skiing. Variations of each of these activities may be most suitable to individuals, but whatever exercise is chosen must conform to the criteria discussed in the previous paragraph. You may combine the activities, doing one one day and another the next, though you need a higher degree of fitness to be able to gain a comparable benefit from combinations of exercises than from one.

CYCLING, ROWING, SKIING, RUNNING: AT HOME

Bicycling, rowing, and cross country skiing require more apparatus and preparation and place greater demands on time and location than the other activities. These problems can be somewhat overcome, for those who wish to pursue it, by buying home, indoor, stationary exercise equipment that simulates the stress of the activity. For those who need or wish to exercise indoors, these are good alternatives. For those who tolerate exercise best if weight bearing is not required, the stationary bicycle may be the best choice.

An additional form of indoor exercise equipment that satisfies the needs of some people is the elastic jogging platform. These small trampolines that sit a few inches above the floor allow walking, running, or jump-rope or dance-like movements against an elastic surface. Avoidance of inclement weather or other threats of the out-of-doors make use of these platforms a good part-time substitute for those who walk or run regularly. The problem with this apparatus is that the energy of the elastic provides a lot of movement, so using the trampoline creates a feeling of more exercise than is actually being done. Pulse or breathing rate need to be monitored to see that sufficient effort is being expended.

SWIMMING

Swimming may be used for muscle strengthening, for general fitness, or for both. The effort for strengthening requires bursts of near maximum effort which, if done properly, could not be sustained for long enough to serve as a fitness exercise. Fitness, conversely, requires prolonged, sustained effort. The strokes may be the same, but the intensity and duration of effort are different.

Swimming is excellent fitness activity if the effort is continuous. You cannot stop for breaks at the end of the pool or interrupt the exercise with any sort of rest. Though it may be possible to sustain the effort for only a few minutes when first starting, the goal to maintain fitness is more than 30 minutes of continuous moderately stressful effort at each workout.

The neck stress of breath-taking from prolonged effort at free style swimming can be avoided by using a snorkel and goggles so the head is kept beneath the water.

Breast-stroking requires a lot of neck extension, lumbar lordosis, and rapid shifts in low back position. Side arm (elementary) back-stroke, while not a competitive swim stroke, places least stress on the low back. It is the best stroke for those with neck or back pain who are working into swimming as a fitness activity.

The biggest problems with swimming as a fitness activity are its seasonal nature and finding regular access to a pool where uninterrupted distance swimming is possible. Remember, to gain full benefits from a fitness program, you must exercise at least every other day. Consequently, most people who include distance swimming in their fitness program use it as a supplemental exercise and depend upon one of the more easily accessible activities for their regular fitness workouts.

To be satisfactory for fitness exercise, swimming pools require a long enough straightaway, with depth to allow swimming laps back and forth without stopping. To be satisfactory for water flexibility and strengthening exercise, swimming pools need to have a standing surface where water is at chest level and arm holds are available on the sides.

AEROBIC DANCING AND CALISTHENICS

Aerobic dancing and calisthenics, with or without music, in groups or alone, are much-publicized and often-attempted means of fitness. The term "aerobic dancing" is used here to mean any dance-type exercise activity that may be done for prolonged periods of time without progressive loss of breath.

Dancing and calisthenic forms of exercises certainly have some great advantages. Most communities have professionals who will lead groups through these types of fitness programs at reasonable cost. The use of music or rhythmic chanting makes exercise more pleasant for some. The social aspects of group activity and the encouragement you get from fellow exercisers may be big pluses.

Most programs can be easily adapted to home use, so you don't need to be with the group on days when you would rather exercise at home alone.

You must take some precautions if one of the variations of aerobic dancing or calisthenics is to be your fitness activity. Most leaders of these groups are exceptionally fit and physically capable people who have and can generate a lot of enthusiasm for exercising. It is very easy for them to lead their followers to push beyond the level for which they are ready. You must remind yourself that what you are seeking is lifetime fitness and that, though you want to steadily progress, pushing too fast is not worth the risk of injury or discouragement.

Another problem with aerobic dancing is that the action may be non-continuous. Aerobic means that you do not get "out of breath" during the activities. In fact, if you are exercising properly, your breathing effort increases so that you are breathing faster and deeper than you normally would. Your breathing does not increase to the point where you feel you have no reserve and must slow way down or stop. You want to reach a plateau where you are breathing deeper and faster than normal, but where, with an effort, you can continue throughout without slowing down the exercise. If the exercises are done with an effort so that you become breathless during one exercise and then stop and "catch your breath" before going to the next, you are not gaining the sort of general fitness benefit discussed here. Aerobic dancing and calisthenics can be easily tailored to provide smooth and rapid transition from one activity to the next without sudden bursts and rests. That is the way this exercise should be done for the results you are seeking.

Aerobic dance exercises may tend to be "ballistic." The rhythm, the music, and the enthusiasm to stay with the group may induce you to make jerking efforts to complete each movement. This jerking is more likely to produce muscle injury. You should be careful to keep your breathing relaxed without breath-holding strains and keep the muscular effort smooth.

If you stay away from these pitfalls and make sure that none of them result in depriving you of the full benefit of a fitness program or lead you to injury, the music, the companionship, the variety of movements, and the adaptability of this form of fitness program may make it the most desirable.

WALKING–JOGGING–RUNNING

By far, the most popular general fitness activity is some variation of jogging. Whether it be walking, jogging, or speed running depends on the level of fitness and experience of the participant.

For those unaccustomed to regular exercise lasting 30 minutes or more without break, the thought of running for that long may sound very unappealing. It does not have to be unpleasant.

The reason running is selected more than any other form of fitness exercise is because of its simplicity. Running requires very little equipment and very little need to compromise for location or weather. The exercise can be done almost any time it can be fitted into the day, so it requires little planning or preparation.

Not only is jogging the fitness activity selected by the most people, but it is the activity that most people stick with. That is, more people who have shown that they accept fitness as a lifetime commitment, by continuous adherance to an exercise program for a year or more, do it by jogging than by any other activity.

Many people know they need to commit to a fitness program but, because they are unfamiliar with it, are reluctant and a little afraid. They may try to satisfy themselves that they have made an effort by buying some equipment or outfits or enrolling in a course or group. Those things are all right but they don't give you what you need. You need commitment and dedication to persist through the fears and some unpleasant aspects of exercising. That is the hard but simple concept. Those who accept it frequently choose the simplest activity, which is jogging.

Some people have back or neck conditions that make prolonged weight-bearing exercise undesirable. An alternative exercise may have to be selected in some cases, but many people who believed they would never be able to run for exercise because of a back or neck condition have been surprised at their successes. Many who have begun with an alternative exercise have switched to running as they developed confidence.

Many people believe from their personal experience, and many people will tell you, that running is very unpleasant. There are times when you misjudge and push too hard at anything and those times are unpleasant, but running does not have to be unpleasant.

Becoming breathless is unpleasant. Feeling nauseous is unpleasant. Having stomach cramps is unpleasant. Those are symptoms of pushing beyond the level of fitness. They do not have to be and should not be common features of a running-for-fitness program.

The mistake made by almost everyone who finds running unpleasant, who gets hurt or sick from running, or who gets discouraged with it is that too much is done too soon. These are foolish, pointless errors that make your fitness project unpleasant and result in lack of progress.

You want to always be making very gradual progress. You want to think in terms of months rather than days. If you are doing very slightly better than you were last month, that is just right. If you have not been on a fitness program before, whether you know it or not, you have been getting very gradually worse in your cardiorespiratory ability each month for all of your adult life. If you have reversed the direction of those changes, you have done a great thing. Your job is to keep the direction of your fitness toward improvement, never to let it turn around the other way again. The rapidity of the progress is not important. If you get discouraged or hurt and quit, your state of fitness will turn direction and start getting worse. So don't take chances—keep the progress very slow, keep it pleasant, keep it safe, but keep it going.

Most people who are not already running for exercise should begin a jogging fitness program by walking. Walk a distance that is very mildly stressful for you—more than you would walk at one time during the ordinary day, but a distance that you are quite sure you can walk without having pain and stiffness afterward. Do gentle flexibility exercises right before and more vigorous ones afterward. Note the distance and the time it took you. Walk at a comfortable pace. Don't try to hurry, but remember that these exercise periods are to be uninterrupted, so don't stop to rest or talk. If you wish, have someone walk with you. Even after you work up to running, you will want to have enough breathing reserve to be able to talk while you run.

For most people, every other day fitness sessions work best. If you have the time and wish to, you can exercise every day and perhaps progress a little faster. Both the good and bad effects of fitness exercise add up, though, so you must be more careful not to hurt yourself if you exercise every day. Even on an every other day schedule, you must remember that you can do far more *once* than you can do regularly. You should not try to increase your level of exercise until you have demonstrated for at least a week that you can maintain your present level without pain and unpleasantness.

So, for at least the first week, continue to take the same walk you took the first day. If, after that time, you are suffering no ill effects from the walking, increase the distance a little. Never make sudden dramatic increases. At any level of fitness, it is not advisable to increase your exercise total for the week by more than 10 percent.

This means that if you walk one mile at each session the first week, you should increase to only about 1.1 mile at each session the second week. Another way of increasing effort which enables you to add variety to the sessions is to add the extra effort on to just one or two sessions. For example, if you walked one mile for each of the first four sessions, you could walk the next four at 1.0, 1.2, 1.0, and 1.2, thus only increasing by 10 percent over the week, but adding an occasional longer effort. Keep some balance, though—don't ever try to do the whole week's effort in one day.

Once you have progressed to the point where you can walk three miles at each session without unpleasantness and painful aftereffects, you are ready to begin to increase your speed. Take a watch for a few days and check the time it takes you to walk three miles at the comfortable pace you have been using. If you are walking over the same course at the same effort, you will find that the times are fairly constant.

Once you have found the predictable, average time that three miles takes you, begin to try to beat that time. Fifteen to 30 seconds faster is plenty of improvement. Don't try to cut more time off at each session. Establish a new pace that you hold for a week or so without unpleasant side effects. Then drop the time again.

Keep lowering the time each week. If you get sore muscles, ease off and just try to stay even for a while and then start up again with the progress. Be sure to carefully stretch any sore muscles each session. If one spot is consistently troublesome, put ice wrapped in towels on it for 20 to 30 minutes after each exercise.

Once you have gotten the time that it takes for you to cover the three miles so low that you feel you cannot walk any faster, you are ready to begin running. The difference between running and walking is that with running, for an instant neither foot is in contact with the ground, whereas walkers always have some contact. Running, of course, allows you to get there faster, though some folks walk faster than others can run. In fact, you can learn to walk very rapidly, but at a certain point picking up speed by running is less effort than trying to walk faster. Your body will tell you when you have reached that point and that is when you should begin to run a portion of the distance.

PRECAUTIONS ABOUT FITNESS EXERCISE

If you proceed with a very gradually increasing fitness schedule such as the one suggested here, the precautions are pretty well built into the program. Of course, people with heart disease or other serious illness that might limit exercise tolerance should obtain their doctor's blessing before beginning any fitness program.

Two commonly used methods monitor the level of stress that an exercise is producing. The simpler, though less exact, is to monitor breathing stress. Breathing should be definitely deeper and more rapid than normal but not so much so that conversation cannot be maintained. If you are breathing so hard that you cannot talk comfortably, you need to slow down.

The other method requires that the pulse be taken. This can be done in the usual way at the wrist. While exercising, counting the "carotid" pulse in the front of the neck may be easier. Subtract your age from 220 and then take 75 percent of that to obtain the "target pulse." For example, if you are 40: 220 minus 40 equals 180 times .75 = 135. This is the rate at which maximum safe fitness is being obtained. If the rate is above that, you are going too fast; if below, you could afford to pick it up a little bit.

These monitors of stress are most often used by those who are well along with a fitness program and are trying to keep their progress going as fast as they safely can. When you are first starting, many physical and psychological factors are not accounted for by these monitoring methods. The beginner does best to stay within the limits imposed by these methods, but not to push hard to maintain a target pulse right at first. If the pulse gets too fast, you must slow down; but if the pulse is lower than the target pulse, don't worry about it until you have accommodated to the exercise. Just keep trying, keep things going in the right direction without injury, and don't worry, at first, about the speed of progress.

chapter seventeen
EXERCISE SUMMARY

These discussions of various forms of exercise may seem overwhelming. No one who has many other things to do could do all these exercises, you may think. There is some truth in that, but consider several things that may relieve your anxieties about exercise.

Very few people do all these exercises all the time. Learning them and working into the usefulness of them takes more time and effort than the regular maintenance. As you do the exercises, you will find what you need to work on the most and can concentrate your effort on what is most effective.

People successfully maintain exercise programs without going through all of every routine every day. Flexibility exercises take a few minutes in morning and evening and a few seconds periodically throughout the day. The general fitness sessions require about an hour every other day and can be done morning, noon, or night as convenient. Follow the general fitness exercise with flexibility exercises. The strengthening exercise can be done on the days that general fitness is not done. The relaxation exercises take some extra time to learn at first but, once learned, can be worked into the day whenever they seem to be needed. Few people on a maintenance program spend more than an hour a day doing exercises.

Most of all, you will find, once into exercising, that you have more time for the rest of your life even if you are investing an hour a day in exercise. If you feel better, can concentrate better on your other tasks, spend less time in hospitals and doctors' offices, spend less time unable to do what you want because you are down, and require less sleep, you will find that when you used to think you "didn't have time for exercise," you were losing your chance for more time to be happy and productive.

chapter eighteen
ANATOMY

The neck must provide the strength to keep the head upright while allowing it to twist, lean, and nod. While so doing, the neck must provide protective passage for the spinal cord to the trunk and limbs, for nerves to the arms, for organs of breathing, talking, and swallowing, and for the major vessels to and from the head. It is expected to do all this and more over a lifetime of stresses.

Details of how stress affects the structure of the neck, how the neck is constructed to withstand those stresses, and how those stresses are distributed through the neck are still being discovered. The anatomical structure, the chemical makeup, and the effects of stress and movement are all different for different people. They all change every day through one person's lifetime and even undergo cyclic changes within the same day. Advances in technology and understanding are constantly providing new ways to look at the structures, determine the chemical composition, or apply engineering principles to analysis of the movements and stresses. With so many different ways to look at so many different things, all of which change all of the time, it is not hard to understand that mysteries of the structure and workings of the neck are still waiting to be discovered.

The scaffold upon which the neck is built is composed of interconnected segments of bone. Living bone is not a china- or ivory-like substance like it appears in museum specimens or frozen meats. Living bone is composed of fibers of a protein, collagen, woven and stranded together and laced with deposits of crystals composed of calcium and other minerals. In the thick outer cortex, the collagen fibers are densely packed together. In the thinner, lacier "marrow" portions of bone, they are more loosely packed. Through all portions of the bone, blood courses, providing oxygen and minerals to sustain living bone cells and allowing the crystals to remake themselves maintaining strength and balance.

The bones are bound together by ligaments. Ligaments are rope-like structures composed of fibers of collagen woven and stranded together. They anchor into the bone by intimately bonding and interweaving with the collagen structure of the bone. The ligaments in their normal state do not contain mineral crystals although bone or "calcium deposits" may form in them as a result of injury repair or repeated stress.

Most ligaments, like a woven rope, have a little "slack" built into the weave, but little true elasticity. They serve as check-reins against excessive motion of the bones and maintain the bones in their normal relationship to one another.

The places where bones interconnect are called joints. Joints vary greatly in shape, composition, and function. The spine contains some unique joints that are quite different from one another and have some features unlike the joints in the arms and legs.

Each separate bone of the neck is called a cervical vertebra. Humans, as do almost all mammals (even the giraffe and the bulldog) have seven of them (see Figure 15). The top one, a ring-shaped bone called the atlas, connects to the skull above and connects below to the second cervical vertebra, called the axis. The seventh cervical vertebra connects to the highest, or first, thoracic vertebra. The 12 thoracic vertebrae are separate, interconnected vertebrae much like the cervical vertebrae above them and the lumbar vertebrae below them, except that the thoracic vertebrae have ribs attached to them.

Except for the first two cervical vertebrae, each two adjacent vertebrae connect directly with each other on the back (posterior) side by a paired set of joints, the facet joints. In front, they make contact and are supported by a complex, specialized joint called the intervertebral disc.

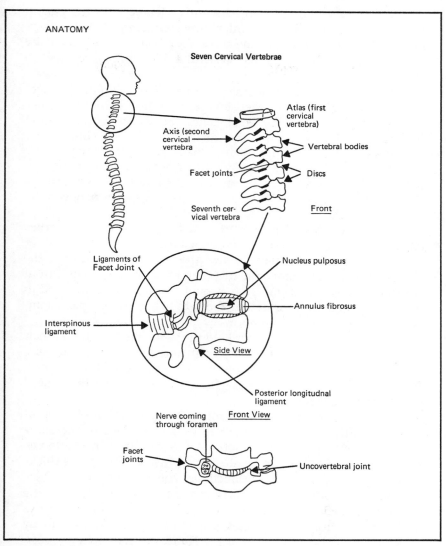

Figure 15   Anatomy

141

The combination of two adjacent vertebrae with the pair of facet joints and the disc that interconnects them is called a "segment." The segments and the discs they include are named by naming the vertebrae such as "cervical 4-5," often abbreviated to "C4-5."

Each vertebra forms a ring of bone around a central space. When the vertebrae are locked together by the joints, the spaces line up forming a tunnel or canal, called the vertebral canal. In the cervical portion of the spine, the canal is filled by the spinal cord, the fluid (cerebro-spinal fluid) that surrounds it, and a membrane sac (meninges) that holds the fluid. At each vertebral segment, one pair of nerves comes out of the sac, passes a short distance through the vertebral canal, and then goes out through spaces between the side walls of the vertebrae.

The spaces between the vertebrae through which the nerves pass are called "foramina," each one being called a "foramen" or an "intervertebral foramen." After the nerves exit through the foramen, many of them join together to form a "plexus" from which separate nerves emerge to provide control of muscles and to bring back sensory information about touch, position, pain, temperature, pressure, and vibration.

Besides the ligaments that hold the vertebrae together at their joints, additional ligaments pass from one vertebra to the next, attaching at connecting points on the vertebrae called "processes." These are guy wires and check-reins and cannot actively control the movement of the spine.

The active control of movement, the proper fine tuning of posture, and the protection of the inactive portions of the spine from excessive stress are the jobs of the muscles. The vertebrae have muscle attachments on all sides. Muscles of various thicknesses and lengths pass in all directions. The muscles provide these functions, not only from one vertebra to another, but also for the whole combined, attached structure of the neck, as it must relate to the head and chest. The muscles function for the neck, not only by direct attachment to the cervical vertebrae, but indirectly by positioning the chest, shoulders, and lower back.

The large muscles that determine the appearance of the neck cover smaller muscles that span shorter distances. The "trapezius" muscles cover the back of the neck down to the shoulder blades. In front, the "sternocleidomastoid" muscles are the long, thick, tubular muscles that stand out when the head is turned. Beneath the sternocleidomastoids are smaller muscles, the "scalenes," that run close to the spine and in close contact with the major nerves that emerge from the spine on their way to the arms. The "rhomboids" are the major group of muscles that pull the scapulae back toward the midline of the back. Numerous other muscles contribute to neck function, but their names are not as commonly known because they are not as large, as visible, or as often named in describing medical problems of the neck.

We know that muscle weakness, muscle stiffness, and loss of muscle function are very important contributors to back and neck pain. Doctors are not often able to zero in on some one spot in some one muscle to locate the source of trouble. Most likely, neck pain actually doesn't occur that way very often. Also, the diagnostic means are not available to really pinpoint muscle problems accurately.

The same difficulty with precision applies to most ligament problems. Many ligaments function in many different ways under different circumstances, and in intimate relationships to the muscles that are all around them. One single point in one single ligament will not likely, by itself, cause persisting neck pain. Even if such a cause were likely, the diagnostic means to prove it is not available.

Doctors who deal with patients with neck pain have means to be reasonably accurate in saying that a neck condition is related to muscle or ligament problems. They cannot, however, often be precise about pinpointing a ligament or muscle, finding exactly what is wrong with it, and determining how long it is going to take the structure to recover.

INTERVERTEBRAL DISC

Some common causes of neck pain often do lend themselves to very precise identification. Many of these involve abnormalities that occur in the intervertebral disc.

The intervertebral disc is a complicated anatomic structure. Though its overall shape may be somewhat like a tiddly-wink, its makeup is anything but a single, predictable material.

The disc is located between the top of the body of one vertebra and the bottom of the body of the vertebra above it. The body of the vertebra is the largest part of the vertebra and is located in the front (anterior) portion of the spine. The back of the vertebral body makes up the front wall of the vertebral canal. The body is somewhat like a baked biscuit in that all the outside surface of it is thicker, more densely packed bone, whereas the central "marrow" portion is spongier.

The outermost portion of the disc is a ligament, passing from the edges of the hard, peripheral rim of the body above to that below. It forms a complete ring. It is a multi-layered woven structure composed somewhat like the tough weave of an automobile tire.

The fibers all insert into and blend with the crystal-laden fibers of the bone above and below. This entire ring of ligament, completely surrounding the space between two adjacent vertebral bodies, is called the "annulus fibrosus." It makes up the outer portion of an intervertebral disc. This ring is a very tough structure which, for most people, survives a lifetime of extraordinary stresses.

The center of each disc is called the "nucleus pulposus." Its chemical content and even its gross physical properties change throughout life and vary within a single day. Its molecules have a high capacity to attract and hold water. They therefore tend to form a gel-like substance.

This central nucleus pulposus and the surrounding rim of annulus fibrosus do not have a distinct border between them as in, say, a jelly donut. Rather, they gradually blend together. The outer layers of the annulus are almost all tough, dense, collagen fibers. The inner layer contains some of the gel-like molecules. Some collagen fibers extend in toward the center so that there are some fibers throughout, though, generally, the closer to the center, the smaller the number of fibers.

The nucleus pulposus is held by walls of annulus fibrosus and by a ceiling and floor composed of the bone of the vertebral bodies above and below. This portion of the bone of the body is called the "chondral plate" or "end plate." The chondral plate is covered on the side of the nucleus by cartilage, the smooth, less brittle material that you observe on joint surfaces at the ends of bones. The cartilage surface blends into the fibers of the inner portion of the annulus and the nucleus.

The content of the nucleus changes throughout life. It gradually loses its capacity to hold water and gradually becomes less gel-like and more fibrous. Although this is a normal life process, this change is called "degeneration" of the disc.

The nucleus of an adolescent or young adult may be about the consistency of a raw oyster; that of middle-age, about that of a boiled shrimp; and in older people, the nucleus becomes more gristly.

The water content of a young, healthy nucleus pulposus may be as high as 88 percent. The disc will follow some of the physical properties of a liquid. One is Pascal's Law, written in the 17th century. The law states that a force anywhere on a contained liquid is transmitted, undiminished, throughout that liquid. This explains why the disc can act as a good shock absorber, keeping the vertebrae apart and the annulus ligaments taut. You can see, also, that if the container has a weakened area, forces will continue to be exerted against it as long as the nucleus remains liquid and remains contained.

As discs lose their water content, they also become smaller. This allows the vertebrae to settle closer together. Discs actually lose some water content through the day and replenish it at night; so if you measure very accurately, you will observe that you are slightly shorter in the evening than you are in the morning. The disc is a little "swollen" in the early morning compared to its state later in the day. The water content is almost, but not entirely, replaced at night, so that very slowly, over a lifetime, the discs lose volume. That is the reason that people become shorter as they age.

All discs degenerate. That much is normal. For some people, one or more discs may degenerate more completely long before their other discs or at a younger age than for other people. This early or rapid degeneration of a disc is sometimes, though most often not, explained by specific injury. The degeneration sometimes, though often not, is associated with pain or other symptoms. Many times, evidence of degeneration is observed on x-rays taken for other reasons in people who are not having neck pain.

VERTEBRAL CANAL AND FORAMINA

The settling together of vertebrae that occurs as a result of disc degeneration results in some decrease in the spaces between the vertebrae at the sides where the nerves exit—the foramina get smaller. For most people, this never matters. Most foramina are big enough so that, even though some room is lost, there is still plenty for the nerve. Not everyone is always so fortunate.

The foramen is formed in front by the vertebral body and disc. Above and below are the side walls of the vertebral canal, called the "pedicles." In back are the "facets." The back roof of the vertebral canal is formed by bony parts of the vertebra called "laminae" and the central backward protruding "spinous process" that can be seen and felt through the skin of thin people. The laminae are more narrow than the body of the vertebra, so there are spaces between the back sides of the adjacent vertebrae. These spaces are occupied by ligaments of unusual elasticity, the "yellow ligaments" or "ligamenta flava."

At the outer corners of the vertebral canal where the laminae that form the roof meet the pedicles that form the sidewalls, processes protrude up and down on both sides of each vertebra. These processes are the "facets" and they join with the facets of the vertebrae above and below like clasped hands, forming the "facet joints."

These facet joints lie right over the foramina where the nerves pass through. Movement occurs in these facet joints and stresses are transmitted through them. In response to stress, the facets may slowly enlarge, forming bone spurs or "osteophytes." The clasped hand relationship may also slowly give so that the facets overlap more than normally. Enlargement and excess overlapping of the facets may further narrow the foramen.

In the cervical spine, the end plates are concave, forming a small hollow that the nucleus occupies. Near the edges, the plates have ridges which, with a little wear and tear on the annulus that connects them, come into contact and take on some of the characteristics of joints. These areas are called the "uncovertebral joints" (also called the "joints of vonLuschka" or the "lateral interbody joints"). Thickening of these ridges, since they form part of the inside wall of the foramen, also may contribute to narrowing of the foramen.

When combined, disc narrowing and degeneration, facet enlargement, and thickening of the bones at the uncovertebral joints may narrow a foramen enough to pinch a nerve. This may occur in people who happen to be born without as much reserve room in their foramina. Foramina, like noses and feet, are bigger in some people than in others.

A term frequently used when discussing problems with a canal or foramen is "stenosis." Stenosis means narrowing of a tubular structure. Stenosis of the vertebral canal would put pressure on the spinal cord as it passes through the neck to the rest of the body. Stenosis of a foramen may put pressure on a nerve where it comes through the spine on its way to the arm. The problems created are very different. The term "stenosis" by itself tells us nothing of the problem except that the cause is related to narrowing of a passageway. Confusion is caused if the term is used as though it described a specific disease or symptom pattern.

BAD DISCS

Tearing or wearing away of the annulus fibers near the uncovertebral joints may result in enough weakening of the supporting ring to allow some of the central nucleus to move toward the periphery, in the direction of the nerve. This sometimes results in more inflammation and thickening with a gradually increasing tendency to pinch the nerve.

Bulging of the annulus and movement of nucleus material into the area of the bulges, like a tire tube with a blistered area, poses the threat of a blow-out or rupture. If this occurs, the fragment of nucleus may move out into the foramen and the pain pattern may change, depending on where and how the nerve is irritated.

The movement of nucleus material into the foramen, whether by a bulge or rupture, diminishes the size of the foramen and crowds the nerve root. Depending on the size of the foramen to begin with and the size of the disc fragment, the movement may narrow the foramen enough to pinch the nerve and cause symptoms.

In some instances, a relatively large piece of the nucleus pulposus may move abruptly through weakened portions of the annulus and produce a sudden onset of pain and loss of function in the nerve that it approximates. The trouble this causes is similar in many ways to that caused by more gradual pinching of the nerve by a narrowed foramen, but the symptoms may be more acute and less responsive to first aid measures.

The amount of movement, the stresses applied, and the shapes and strength of the various structures all vary at each segment. The segments with the greatest curvature bear the greatest amount of shear stress—the tendency of one bone to slide down on the other The annulus and the ligaments of the facet joints must resist these stresses. The lower segments of the cervical spine where the curvature is greatest and the shear stress highest are where trouble most often occurs from narrowed foramina and bad discs. Maintaining the head back over the shoulders reduces this shear stress (see Figure 16).

Experiments have shown that simply pinching a nerve root does not usually cause all the symptoms that people have from bad discs. Perhaps some of the chemicals involved in the degeneration process of the nucleus escape and irritate the nerve. Perhaps the body's attempt to repair the annulus causes inflammation and scarring of the nerve. Perhaps some of the symptoms come from small branches of the nerve in the area rather than from damage to the large nerve root. People who have many symptoms likely have some combination of these factors.

The practice of explaining symptoms by identifying the site of difficulty is not an exact science. The source of certain pain patterns and patterns of nerve dysfunctions can be traced to this area where the disc is in proximity to the nerve root with more confidence and precision than can the sources of other common spinal disorders. When these specific patterns of pain and dysfunction exist, physi-

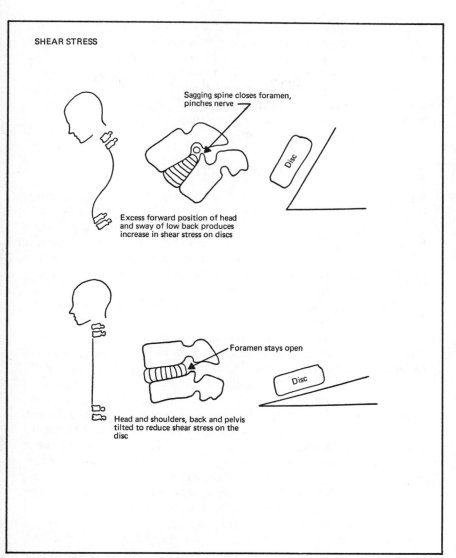

Figure 16 Shear Stress

cians experienced in evaluating these disorders can predict with a high degree of accuracy the spot of origin of the trouble. This accuracy can be further improved by using x-ray techniques. The most widely used technique, the myelogram, requires placing a contrast material (dye) into the spinal fluid, outlining the vertebral canal. Disc bulging or rupture will usually be seen as a failure of formation of the full outline of the canal.

SURGICAL TREATMENT

Surgical treatment for neck conditions is usually considered when pain is so severe, is so prolonged, or is both that the risks and uncertainties of an operation are considered worth taking. Other factors, such as loss of feeling and loss of muscle power from a pinched nerve in the neck, are important considerations in deciding about surgery, but pain is usually the problem that leads the patient to consider surgery.

Most neck pain problems would not be helped by surgery. Many of those that would be helped by surgery would also eventually get just as much better without the surgery. This leaves a relatively small group of people with a problem that has a surgical remedy and that is causing so much trouble that waiting it out with nonsurgical treatment is no longer tolerable.

The great majority of neck pain problems that do have a surgical remedy are those that involve irritation of a nerve where it passes through the foramen. Here the nerve is bordered by facets that may be enlarged by bone spurs (osteophytes) caused by wear and tear changes or injury. The nerve turns around the edge of the body of the vertebra right where the ridges along the edges form the "uncovertebral joints," a site where osteophytes commonly form. This is the site also where the nucleus of the disc commonly bulges or ruptures through the annulus.

If symptoms call for surgical treatment and the physician can localize the source of the difficulty to the spot described in the previous paragraph, an operation can be done with reasonably predictable success. The physician's analysis can usually lead to a conclusion about the exact location of the difficulty and the source of the problem; that is, the analysis can determine whether a disc fragment has suddenly ruptured or the nerve is pinched by a slowly enlarging bone spur.

The operation usually includes removal of some or all of the nucleus portion of the disc. It may also include an attempt to fuse the two vertebrae of the involved segment together.

This spot is near the center of several vital structures: the spinal cord, the vertebral and carotid arteries, the jugular vein, the trachea, and the esophagus. These structures cannot be safely cut through or widely moved about. Therefore, widely exposing this spot so that the surgeon can work around all sides of it at the same time is not possible.

Two surgical approaches to this area are commonly used. The decision about what approach is to be used depends upon factors derived from the patient's symptoms and findings and upon the experience and preference of the surgeon.

One approach is through a longitudinal (up and down) incision in the middle of the back of the neck. The muscles are separated at their attachments to the middle of the spine on the side of the problem. The nerve is exposed by removing part of the facets. Any ruptured nucleus material next to the nerve can also be removed. The operation is sometimes called a "foraminotomy" since it enlarges the foramen.

All operations on the back of the neck are sometimes called, not always correctly, cervical "laminectomies." Technically, the term should only be used for operations in which the lamina is removed, but the term is often used in a more general sense to refer to any of several operations done in this area.

Operations on the back of the neck for fusion only, without removal of anything, are sometimes done to strengthen a neck rendered unstable by injury to the bones.

The other approach taken for the common need for neck surgery, nerve irritation at the foramen, is the anterior (front of the neck) approach. The incision is usually transverse (crosswise) though it may be slanted up and down on one side. The surgeon comes to the middle, deep in the neck, before moving to the side of the symptoms so that the incision may or may not be on the same side of the neck as the symptoms. Most of the disc is removed at the involved segment, the approach to the site of the problem being through the disc space. The space may be left open, filled with bone from a bone bank, or filled with a bone graft taken from the patient's hip, depending upon the specific circumstances of the problem and the surgeon's preference.

SPONDYLOSIS

The combination of disc degeneration and bone thickening with spur formation is sometimes called "spondylosis." Spondylosis occurs to some extent in everyone and is usually not symptomatic. As previously explained, symptoms may occur if these degenerative processes lead to pinching one of the nerves.

If the bone thickening and enlargement of spurs is severe, it may narrow the vertebral canal. This may be especially troublesome for people whose canals were smaller than average to begin with. This combination makes these people particularly susceptible to spinal cord damage from neck injuries that would otherwise not have been serious. Bone thickening and enlarged spurs may also cause slowly progressive loss of cord function from the pinch produced by stenosis of the canal. This spinal cord damage, which can cause paralysis and loss of normal sensation, is called spondylotic myelopathy.

SYMPATHETIC NERVES AND
VERTEBRAL ARTERIES

The sympathetic nervous system is a body-wide network of nerves that provides fine adjustments of blood flow and other body functions that depend upon "tone." We don't have direct conscious control over our sympathetic nervous system, though it is closely in tune with our emotions and activities involving such things as blood pressure, heart and breath rate, sweating, pupil size, and skin temperature.

Important centers of the sympathetic nervous system are located along the side of the cervical spine. The branches travel in rich supply along blood vessels of the neck. Local blood flow and muscle tone in the eyes, ears, and throat may be influenced by the sympathetic structures in the neck.

The vertebral arteries, major suppliers of blood to the brain, pass through holes in the transverse processes of the sixth through the second cervical vertebrae. Changes in shape, position, or function of these vertebrae can influence flow in the vertebral arteries or tone in the sympathetic nerves that accompany the arteries.

The presence of these structures in the neck and their anatomic intimacy with the cervical spine provide an anatomic explanation of how such symptoms as dizziness, blurred vision, ringing in the ears, changes in voice or swallowing, and localized patterns of changes in skin temperature or tone *can* be related to abnormalities in the neck. Such symptoms have many other causes, so often a neck condition is completely unrelated, or just partially related, to such problems.

SHOULDER ANATOMY

Shoulder movement occurs at two joints, both controlled by several muscles.

The shoulder blade (scapula) glides forward (protracts) and backward (retracts) across the chest wall. The upper arm moves on the scapula at a ball and socket joint. The two joints usually move together during ordinary activities.

The major nerves and blood vessels that arise from the neck and chest pass into the arm beneath the shoulder joint, through the arm pit (axilla). The folds that form the axilla are composed in front by the large pectoral muscles from the chest and in back by the latissimus dorsi, very wide muscles sweeping up from the lower and mid-back to insert on the upper arm. The contour of what, externally, is seen as the shoulder is rounded out by the deltoid muscle, which is what you grab if you reach across the body with one hand to grasp the opposite shoulder.

Deep to these large, visible muscles is a group of muscles that starts at the shoulder blade and wraps its tendons around the top of the humerus (bone of the upper arm). Because they control shoulder rotation and because their tendons form a "cuff" around the top of the humerus, these muscles are called the "rotator cuff." They must work through a very wide range of motion, under cramped circumstances and often under great stress. These muscles commonly become inflamed, producing "rotator cuff tendinitis."

chapter nineteen
NECK-RELATED
MEDICAL PROBLEMS

Neck pains, as we have seen, often result from many factors. With the neck being so central to the function of the body and the anatomy of the neck so filled with vital structures, understanding how the neck can cause pain or dysfunction in other parts is easy.

Neck function is part of a linkage of functions between the head and the body. When the neck fails, parts on either end of that chain may fail. When there is malfunction at either end, failure of the neck is more likely. The more one end fails, the worse the other end functions, completing the "vicious circle."

This close, interdependent relationship between neck functions and other body functions sometimes creates difficulty in telling what went wrong first, or, where the worst, or underlying, malfunction exists. The mind's ability to locate the source of difficulty from where it feels like the pain is coming is not always accurate. Pains may be referred; that is, they may be felt at a site distant from the site of the problem.

These distant, or referred, pains may have several explanations. Irritation of a nerve may cause pain to occur anywhere along the course of that nerve. Interference with function of a distal part by disturbing its blood or nerve supply may cause it to hurt. Referred pain is not always explained by these mechanisms. There exist, in the brain and spinal cord, patterns of awareness of sensation and coordination of body functions which are not fully understood and may be the source of some distant pains.

In this chapter, we want to explore some of the common problems that are *sometimes* related to disorders of the structures of the neck. These symptoms can all occur from other causes. You cannot assume, even when known problems exist in the neck, that these problems are related to the neck problem. Even if medical investigation has provided strong evidence that one of these problems is *related* to the neck problem, saying that the relationship is causal may not be possible; that is, no one may be able to say whether the neck problem causes the other symptoms. Though the existence of such a relationship should never be assumed without supporting medical evidence, these relationships do exist so often that knowledge of them is necessary to an understanding of neck problems.

HEADACHE

Millions of people suffer from headaches. Most headaches are extracranial, meaning they begin outside the skull. Most people who have recurrent headaches have "tension headaches" (also called "muscle-contraction headaches"). These are often related to neck problems.

Rarely, headache reflects a serious internal problem within the head such as brain tumor or meningitis. If the headaches have been present for a long time and are not progressing or changing in character, if they are not accompanied by other serious nervous system disturbances such as memory loss, seizures, changes in vision or other sensory function, or vomiting, and if medical examinations show no evidence of an internal problem, you can be reasonably well assured that the headaches are from some external cause.

Some causes of headache have nothing to do with neck problems. Some people develop headaches from eating meals with high contents of monosodium glutamate (such as in Oriental foods), nitrites (such as in some hot dogs and other cured meat), or foods to which they are sensitive (common ones being chocolate and cheeses). Some people with hypoglycemia (periodic low blood sugar) get headaches in the early morning or when deprived of food for long periods. Withdrawal from caffeine may cause headache in some individuals.

Headache may be a side effect of certain medicines. Paradoxically, headaches can occur with medicines sometimes taken for head and neck pain related problems—the nonsteroidal anti-inflammatory drugs. Steroids (cortisone-like drugs), tetracyclines, vitamin overdose, and many other drugs have also been associated with headache in certain individuals.

Another uncommon form of headache is the "cluster" headache. Cluster headaches usually occur in men between ages 20 and 50. They are present on one side of the head only and are extremely severe, but temporary. They recur, maybe several times within days, and then may disappear for weeks or months.

Migraine headaches are fairly common, though not nearly so common as many people suppose. The term "migraine" has been so often associated with severe headaches that many headache sufferers call their headaches "migraine" because the pain is so severe. Migraine headaches can be very painful, but so can tension headaches. The distinction between the two is not based upon severity of pain and you should not assume a headache is a "migraine" because the pain is severe.

Migraine headaches usually occur on one side of the head only or at least predominantly on one side. Migraine headaches are usually preceded by a drowsy feeling or an uneasy forewarning that the headache is on its way. Migraines become progressively severe over hours to days and may be accompanied by nausea, vomiting, chills, fever, and exhaustion. A minority of migraine sufferers have the "classic" form of migraine, which has the characteristics of visual abnormalities, emotional changes, and a strong family history of the problem.

Tension headaches usually occur on both sides of the head. The pain may be very severe, but tension headaches are not commonly associated with vomiting, nausea, or vision changes. Tension in the muscles of the jaws, temples, forehead, or back of the head and feelings of tightness or pulsations around the head are common.

The underlying cause, or factor, that first sets a tension headache in motion is not always apparent and may not always be the same. The common factor is that the mechanism by which the pain is produced is tension in the muscles of the head and neck.

Fatigue, other illness, nervousness, emotional upset, or posture stress can set off tension states. Sometimes certain activities such as driving, particular tasks at work, or the need to deal with some conflict at home can be identified as a trigger.

Those with occupations requiring prolonged, fairly stationary posture with the head forward and down are commonly afflicted. Secretaries, draftsmen, and machine operators have this problem more frequently than people whose jobs permit more mobility and a more upright posture of the head.

The muscles involved are the muscles of the back of the neck and those of the head. The trapezius muscles from the shoulders up to the sides of the neck and the small muscles along the middle of the back of the neck are held tensely and under increased stress because the head is usually in a forward leaning "attentive" pose. Tender areas in the mid-portion of the trapezius and at the bony knobs at the back of the head where the neck muscles insert onto the skull frequently accompany tension headaches.

If you place your finger just in front of the front attachment of the top of your ear lobe, you can feel a pulsation. This is the temporal artery. It courses through and supplies blood to a broad muscle along the side of the head, the temporal muscle.

The temporal muscle and another flat muscle over the forehead, the frontal muscle, control much of the facial expression of attentiveness. Most people who are tense can be easily recognized to be so because of the subtle changes in facial expression produced by these muscles. A third group of muscles, those controlling the jaw, also contribute to facial expression.

Muscles are meant to contract. Making muscles work makes them healthier and more able to bear stress without pain. Healthy contractions require periods of relaxation, though, and inadequate relaxation is what leads to tension muscle pain.

The difference between healthy, painless muscle function and tension produced muscle pain can be demonstrated by experimenting with the quadriceps muscle, the big muscle at the front of the thigh. These muscles do a great deal of work painlessly, during a long walk. If you stand back to the wall and bend the knees, as when doing a wall slide exercise, after only a matter of seconds these same muscles get uncomfortable. Within a minute or two these muscles, which can walk for long periods, produce severe pain from the sustained tension. Neck and face muscles produce tension pain by the same mechanism.

Treatment for tension headache follows the same principles and most of the same techniques as described for neck pain. The same first aid, posture, psychological care measures, relaxation techniques, and exercises that help neck pain help tension headaches. This similarity is not surprising since many aspects of the problems are the same, and the two conditions frequently coexist.

Some modifications of the application of the technique are needed to provide attention to the muscles of the head.

Facial muscles may be exercised by holding an exaggerated facial expression tightly in an isometric contraction of the muscles. The same technique is used as is described in the section on relaxation exercises. These exercises may make the facial muscles stronger and improve their tone. The contractions are held for progressively longer periods as in doing isometric strengthening exercises. Strength of the small facial muscles may be less important than the awareness of the activity of these muscles that the exercise produces. Once aware of the tension, you may take measures to relax the muscles more easily before the problem becomes painful.

Massage of face, head, and neck muscles works both as a preventative and as first aid treatment for tension headache. A specialized form of massage, acupressure, can also be very useful for many people with tension headaches. The methods to be used for massage and acupressure are discussed in the chapter on first aid.

Some special techniques apply to relieving tension headaches. They may also relieve tension-related neck pain in the absence of headache. You should remember that tension headache is related to the anatomy and function of the neck and that the many recommendations made throughout this book for the control of neck pain also apply to the control of tension headaches.

JAW, TEETH, AND THE T.M.J. SYNDROME

Open your mouth and insert your index finger as far back in the corner of your open mouth as it will go. Place the thumb of the same hand on the outside of the cheek just below the ear lobule and just above the angle of the jaw. Your thumb and index finger now surround small, but extremely strong, muscles.

These muscles are common sites of tension. They provide the mechanism of "gritting your teeth" or "setting your jaw." The tension in these muscles can be seen at the angle of the jaw in some people. The tightness of the internal portion of this muscle group may be felt with the tip of the index finger.

The jaw joins the skull at a joint within and near the top of these muscles, the temporomandibular joint (T.M.J.). Tension in these muscles produces tension across the T.M.J. Problems associated with pain in this area are sometimes called the "T.M.J. Syndrome."

Tension of these muscles tends to hold the teeth clenched together. The extreme of this is actual grinding of the teeth, called "bruxism." Grinding of the teeth that can be heard or seen to be producing damage is a sign of severe tension and is a call for psychological and dental professional assistance.

The T.M.J. Syndrome may follow major dental work or injuries to the jaw. In such cases the primary problem may be from the teeth and the primary care should come from the dentist. Even when such is not the case, severe T.M.J. Syndromes may sometimes be helped by dental appliances or dental reconstruction.

The less severe, and much more common, problem of painful T.M.J. tension and teeth clenching can usually be self-treated by recognition and some simple measures. T.M.J. Syndrome is usually a part of the same problem that includes neck pain and tension headaches. All of the things that apply to treatment of tension related neck pain and headache, therefore, also apply to treatment of the T.M.J. Syndrome. In addition, some special measures help with the T.M.J. Syndrome and, often, consequently help with neck pain and headaches as well.

An essential feature of the treatment of T.M.J. Syndrome is

recognition of the problem. During only one instant should the teeth ever actually be in contact. That is at the moment of swallowing. All the rest of the time, the teeth should be slightly separated. Remember this and see how often, during the times of neck pain, headache, or jaw pain you catch yourself with unnecessary contact of the teeth. The relaxed state of the jaw muscles allows the teeth to separate. By keeping the teeth separated you can help keep jaw and related neck and face muscles relaxed. You may use a pencil or other convenient mouth-bite object to keep teeth apart during leisure time.

Persisting tension in jaw muscles may lead to loss of motion in the temporomandibular joint. The result is inability to open the mouth widely. Just as flexibility exercises on an hourly basis are required to regain lost motion in other joints, repeated efforts to open the mouth as widely as possible may be necessary to regain and maintain jaw motion. When you open your mouth widely, you may feel a stretch and relaxation of other face and neck muscles and the facial skin.

Massage of the jaw muscles between the index finger tip and thumb tip may help relieve tension and assist with flexibility exercises.

These muscles have tremendous strength. Strengthening exercises aren't really necessary, but isometric teeth clenching, in the manner of contrast-relaxation exercises, helps with recognition of the feelings of tightness and relaxation.

SHOULDER TENDINITIS

Pain and restricted motion in the shoulder joint may occur in conjunction with neck pain. The problem often involves inflammation of the cuff of tendons that rotate the shoulder and so may be called "rotator cuff tendinitis."

When speaking of the "shoulder," in this context, we refer to the area around the top of the upper arm—the area you cover with your hand if you place your arm across the chest and grasp the opposite shoulder with your hand. Pain in the muscles near the neck and around the shoulder blade is also sometimes called shoulder pain, but we are considering here a problem involving the immediate area of the shoulder joint.

Whether rotator cuff tendinitis can be caused by neck conditions and whether it can be the cause of neck conditions are controversial points. Both are common problems of the same age group (middle), so their coexistence in certain people may just reflect the tendency of those people to develop structural pain syndromes rather than some causal relationship.

Possible causal links are the role of tension and loss of flexibility. Many factors about rotator cuff tendinitis are unknown. We do know that it almost always, eventually (maybe after years), goes away. The only thing that has been consistently found to prevent progression and to speed recovery is the regular performance of flexibility exercise. Once all the motion is regained, the pain usually disappears.

Whether reflex tension in shoulder muscles from neck conditions, diminished normal use of the shoulder because of tension states and neck pain, or fear of allowing full motion in a shoulder that hurts because of referred pain from the neck can actually cause rotator cuff tendinitis can only be considered and not proven.

The lesson that should emerge from consideration of these facts about shoulder and neck pain is that shoulder motion should be maintained at all costs. Except in very obvious situations, such as broken bones, you are never wise to "rest" the shoulder by keeping it still. Pain in the shoulder means that the shoulder should be moved through its full range several times a day. This does not mean that the shoulder should be subjected to heavy resistance such as lifting weights or to performance of athletic activities requiring sudden jerking, forceful efforts. The shoulder should be rested from those things, but it should be gently moved through its full range.

When testing yourself for shoulder motion, you may have a tendency to "cheat." The arms should come fully next to the ear when reaching overhead for the ceiling. Tilting the head toward the shoulder to get the arm next to the head is cheating. If the arm will not come smoothly and fully overhead to touch the ear with the head straight, you have trouble in the shoulder and it needs flexibility exercises. The same is true if the back of the hand cannot be placed back between the shoulder blades.

The sections of this book that deal with flexibility exercises and with anatomy contain more specific information about the shoulder. The principles of first aid for neck pain also apply to shoulder pain.

CHEST PAIN

The large muscles of the chest wall are controlled by nerves that pass through the neck. These muscles participate in neck and shoulder posture. Chest pain may occur because of tension in these muscles. Chest pain may also occur as referred pain—pain that is stimulated by some disorder in the neck but interpreted by the brain as coming from the chest.

Besides the annoyance, the problem that chest pain presents is the need to be certain it is not occurring as a result of some serious problem from within the chest, heart pain, or angina, being the most common worry.

Heart pains are notoriously hard to interpret. Some people with angina have pain in the arm, some have pain in the neck or jaw, and those with chest pain don't always have the pain occur in the same part of the chest.

One characteristic of angina is that the pain is usually produced by exercise and is rapidly relieved by rest. Angina does not usually involve tenderness, or pain brought on by pressure over the painful areas.

The problem of distinguishing chest pain produced by neck conditions from chest pain brought on by heart or lung conditions is sufficiently difficult that it should be done, in part, by trying to rule out heart and lung conditions. This at least means a consultation with your family doctor and may mean x-rays, cardiograms, stress tests, or consultations with a specialist.

Once you are reassured that nothing is wrong with the heart and lungs, certain chest pains may be properly treated by treating neck and shoulder conditions outlined in this book. Adding push-up exercises to strengthen the muscles of the front of the chest wall may be helpful in some instances.

Often chest pain related to neck problems is not really severe but is merely frightening. The reassurance of passing all of the tests to rule out internal problems and the knowledge that chest pain really does commonly result from neck conditions may be all the "treatment" that is needed.

THORACIC OUTLET SYNDROMES

Once the nerves from the spinal cord pass through the cervical spine, they travel to their destinations in the chest, arm, or hand, protected for the most part by a cushion of muscles. Some sharp turns and some tight spots, however, can cause trouble.

Shortly after leaving the spine most of the nerves join together into a plexus from which single nerves emerge. This joining occurs at the base of the neck and upper part of the arm pit. The nerves and plexus are subjected to stretch from neck and arm positions as they make the turns down and out to shoulder level and then down and in to pass into the arm. The nerves are large at this level and are accompanied by large blood vessels, so the passage is pretty crowded.

If the neck and shoulder muscles are tight, if the shoulder posture is poor, or if the nerves are sensitive from problems elsewhere along their course, symptoms may occur from stretch or pressure upon them as they pass through this outlet from the chest to the arm—the so-called "thoracic outlet syndrome."

An annoying, mildly painful, tingling sensation in the hand and arm is the common symptom from thoracic outlet syndrome. The sensation usually comes and goes and can often be reproduced by certain positions of the head or the arm. Not uncommonly, the sensation will occur at night and awaken you and can be relieved by moving the arm about. The most common site of the tingling is along the little finger side of the hand. Sometimes the pressure is severe enough to pinch off blood flow so the pulse in the wrist diminishes when assuming the position that produces the symptoms.

Thoracic outlet syndromes tend to occur more often in women than in men. Possible explanations are that the breasts cause a downward traction effect that increases tension on the nerves at the outlet, that the chest muscle development and strength is less than in men, and that more women work at occupations that involve prolonged forward, leaning, sitting postures.

Most thoracic outlet syndromes come and go and are not really severe. Once the anxiety created by the symptoms is relieved by an explanation of them, people rarely need to undergo major treatment efforts. Doctors can often accurately determine the site of the pinch from the analysis of the position that causes the problem and can design operations that will relieve the pinched areas. Symptoms severe enough that you would want to have an operation for them are unusual, however.

The thoracic outlet syndromes are treated by adhering to the principles of good posture and exercise outlined in this book. Shoulder retraction and elevation exercises and maintenance of shoulders back and head up posture are particularly important. Large-breasted women with these symptoms should wear extra-support bras.

CARPAL TUNNEL AND OTHER NERVE ENTRAPMENT SYNDROMES

After the nerves to the arms leave the thoracic outlet, they course through muscles except for some sharp turns and tight passages at the elbow and wrist. The site of nerve irritation is not always the same as where the pain or numbness is felt. Sometimes nerve irritation at the elbow or wrist can be felt as pain in the shoulder and neck.

The site of nerve irritation beyond the shoulder that most commonly produces neck and shoulder pain is at the wrist. The median nerve must pass through a tight canal on the underside of the wrist on its way to enter the hand. Pressure on the median nerve in this "carpal tunnel" is a common cause of pain and numbness of the thumb, long, and index fingers, called the "carpal tunnel syndrome." Sometimes the pain from carpal tunnel syndrome radiates up to the neck. Less often, the pain is felt more in the neck than in the hand.

The diagnosis of carpal tunnel syndrome can be confirmed by an electrical test called the nerve conduction test. If the diagnosis is made, treatment of carpal tunnel syndrome, usually by surgical release of the ligaments that hold the nerve in the tunnel, will usually relieve the symptoms. In the unusual cases where the main symptoms of carpal tunnel syndrome are neck pains, carpal tunnel release may cure neck and shoulder pain.

At several other areas in the arm major nerves can be irritated as they pass by joints, or can be entrapped under ligaments or fibrous bands. In very unusual, though occasional, cases a major symptom of such nerve problems is neck pain.

DIZZINESS AND HEARING TROUBLE

The flow of blood to the ear and the portion of the brain with which the ear communicates may depend on neck function. The sympathetic nerves may ·indirectly affect this flow.

Dizziness, a roaring sound, or ringing in one or both ears are symptoms of ear dysfunction that can occasionally be caused by neck disorders.

Movement of the head may produce dizziness and other ear symptoms as a direct result of change in inner ear position. If the head, and with it the ear, are held still and the symptoms are caused by rotating the body so that the neck turns, pressure on the vertebral artery or sympathetic nerves could be the cause of the problem.

This distinction is not always easy to make. Testing by an ear specialist or neurologist can give a more accurate idea of whether a neck disorder may be causing dizziness or ringing in the ears.

Besides dizziness, pressure on the vertebral artery where it passes through the cervical spine may cause so-called "drop attacks"—sudden, brief losses of consciousness. If caused by vertebral artery compression in the neck, these attacks are usually related to rotation and extension of the neck. Such movement of the neck would not ordinarily cause any problem. But if the vertebral arteries are previously abnormal, or other blood flow to the brain impaired, as from arteriosclerosis, the additional pressure from extremes of neck rotation and extension may critically reduce the blood flow to the brain.

THROAT PAIN AND
SWALLOWING TROUBLE

Large bone spurs on the front of the spine may cause direct obstruction to swallowing. This is an unusual occurrence. The possibility can be suggested by a regular x-ray showing the bone spur and may be confirmed by specialized x-rays taken while you are swallowing.

A feeling of incoordination of swallowing and loss of normal feeling at the back of the throat may rarely occur as a result of sympathetic nerve dysfunction from neck disorders.

EYE TROUBLE

Problems with eye function can produce neck pain and, less commonly, can result from neck disorders.

Wearing bifocal glasses may result in uncomfortable posturing of the head and neck to provide adequate vision. Need for proper glasses may lead to a strained, head forward position which may produce tension neck pains.

The pathways of the sympathetic nerves along the side of the cervical spine and along with the arteries that pass through the cervical spine provide an explanation for the unusual occurences of blurred vision, droopy eyelids, or difference in pupil size caused by abnormalities in the neck.

GENERAL DISORDERS, ARTHRITIS,
FIBROMYOSITIS

Many generalized diseases may affect neck function. Any disturbance of nerve or muscle function adversely affects the function of the neck.

Any of the arthritic diseases may produce neck pain. Most people who have been told they have arthritis in the neck, however, don't really have an arthritic disease. Local changes of disc degeneration and bone spurring may produce symptoms from the joints in the neck. These changes may be called arthritis but do not mean that an arthritic disease exists. Such changes are also often called "spondylosis," a term that describes changes seen on x-rays and does not describe the symptoms or possibility of future trouble. The x-ray changes that lead to the terms "arthritis" or "spondylosis" commonly occur in people with no symptoms whatever. Therefore, determining whether these changes, when seen on an x-ray, are related to any symptoms that are present at the time is difficult.

A diagnosis may describe a syndrome or a disease. The difference is that in the case of the syndrome, doctors observe that a combination of abnormalities exists at the same time, but the relationship and common cause of the abnormalities are not understood, whereas in the case of a disease, the underlying cause or the reason for the interrelationship of the abnormalities is known.

A common diagnosis given to many people is that of "fibromyositis." Fibromyositis is more of a syndrome than a disease. Generalized feelings of aching and stiffness, trouble sleeping, chronic fatigue, poor nutrition habits, inadequate exercise, and the occurrence of "trigger spots" of tenderness are the combination of problems that constitutes the fibromyositis syndrome. Which of these factors causes the others and whether some unknown underlying factor causes them all are unknown.

Calling this combination of problems "fibromyositis" may be a convenient way for those who understand to communicate briefly. The practice of using the term, however, may sometimes create a misunderstanding that some known disease exists. The application of this term does not imply understanding of the cause of the problem and does not reduce the need to attack each problem by the self-care measures described in this book. The same applies to the use of such terms as "arthritis" (when used in a nonspecific way that does not describe some known form of arthritis) or "spondylosis."

chapter twenty
BEYOND READING
THIS BOOK

Some things you learn in this book are interesting but don't have much personal application. Some apply personally during this learning process and then diminish in importance. Some apply when your neck hurts and not when it doesn't—they can be tucked away to be pulled out in time of need. Others are of continuous and lasting importance.

Sometimes you too easily let what you have learned slip away, only to slide back into old habits. The challenge now is to find what is in your life to make the important changes permanent.

Very few people have the discipline and drive to maintain difficult changes all alone. Of course, the responsibility and the main energy must come from you. One of the best ways to make sure you fulfill your obligations to yourself is to involve other people. They don't do it for you but they can encourage you. Their help can keep you going through hard times if you know that failing would be not only failing yourself but others.

Your spouse, your family, and those closest to you need to know the details of your struggle and be involved in all phases of it.

Having more casual friends, acquaintances, and co-workers know what you are doing also helps. Boring them with accounts of your symptoms and your difficulties doesn't help you or them, but hearing of your successes inspires them. Everyone is involved in personal struggles and takes inspiration from the success of others, regardless of the problem. Sharing your successes commits you to maintain them. If you get lazy and slack off on your commitment, you risk disappointing others as well as yourself.

One particularly good way to combine the social and personal commitments is to become involved in new group activities that compliment your efforts. YMCA, swim clubs, track clubs, health spas, and dance groups offer exercise programs that combine the benefits of enjoyable forms of exercise with the stimulation and encouragement of group membership. Church, medical or social service organization based encounter groups, discussion groups, or group therapy sessions provide the same thing for the psychosocial aspects of the problem. Union or other workers' organizations, business organizations, or labor-management forums may provide a place to discuss relationships between neck pain and occupational activity.

Beyond yourself, your family, your friends, and your community, things that are wrong with the whole culture make resolving the problems created by neck pain difficult. Careers need to be designed for a lifetime so that adjustments are made in the style of the work for those who can no longer do what they once could. Unions and management need to recognize and push for proper working conditions to prevent excessive neck and back strain. Workers need exercise breaks more than coffee breaks. Most people need exercise at noon a lot worse than they need lunch. Recreation must mean personal involvement and satisfaction and not just watching a few superstars exercise on television. A pervasive attitude exists that health problems are someone else's responsibility—the doctor, the employer, the government, the family. Those attitudes must change and society must pressure people to be well rather than encourage them to be sick.

This culture is full of people who don't exercise enough, who are overweight, who do jobs that are poorly designed, who are ignorant of how to accomplish work efficiently and safely, who don't know how to do anything about it and are afraid to try. The solution has to be education that is understood and practiced. Doing things right yourself is the first step in reaching that solution. When you have finished this book, you will already be ahead of most people. Keep right on going and get all that is in it for you. As you do, teach some others too and push for changes that will make it better for everyone.

GLOSSARY

Abdomen—Portion of the trunk below the chest, above the pelvis, and in front of the spine. Bordered by muscles in front. Contains stomach, intestines, liver, pancreas, and spleen.

Abominal muscles—Muscles that support and form the walls of the abdominal cavity. Extend from the ribs to the pelvis and around to the lumbar spine.

Abduction—Pulling away from the center of the body as in spreading the legs apart or lifting the arm to the side.

Active exercise—Exercise done using only the force of your own muscles with no outside assistance.

Acupressure—Technique of relieving pain by applying deep pressure in specified locations in the muscles.

Adam's apple—Prominence of cartilage around the larynx in the front of the neck.

Adduction—Pulling toward the center of the body as in pulling the legs in to squeeze the knees together or pulling the arm down to the side.

Adjustment—In referring to the spine, usually meant to indicate a positioning of spinal parts to try to correct some malalignment or loss of normal position.

Aerobic dancing—Rhythmic exercise usually done to music. Action is continuous, without rest periods.

Anatomy—Study of the form of the body.

Angina—Pain in the arm, chest, neck, or jaw originating from the heart.

Annulus fibrosus—Outside ring of the intervertebral disc. A ring-shaped ligament attaching to the vertebral bodies above and below and surrounding the nucleus pulposus in its center.

Anterior—Toward the front. As opposed to "posterior," which means toward the back.

Anti-inflammatory—Any drug or other agent (for example, ice) meant to decrease inflammation.

Arc—Portion of a circle. Measure of circular motion.

Arthritis—Anything that results in inflammation of joints. Sometimes imprecisely used to mean anything that causes pain in or around joints or to refer to certain x-ray changes around joints.

Atlas—The highest or first cervical vertebra. The top bone of the spine.

Axis—The second cervical vertebra.

Axilla—The area under the shoulder. Region of the arm pit.

Ballistic exercise—Exercise done by rapidly repeating, "bouncing" efforts.

Biofeedback—Technique of teaching relaxation by using devices to make you more aware of the body's reactions to tension-provoking situations.

Body of vertebra—Large block-shaped portion of a vertebra. Located on the front side of the spine. Also called the "centrum."

Bruxism—Severe and habitual grinding of the teeth.

Calcium deposit—Place where crystals containing calcium occur other than where they normally occur in bone. Usually occur as a response to inflammation or injury.

Carotid—Large arteries in front of the neck.

Carpal tunnel syndrome—Symptoms caused by pressure on the median nerve at the wrist.

Calisthenics—Exercises done in series, usually in rhythm.

Carrying movements—Direct forward-and-back or side-to-side movements at the neck or the waist.

Cartilage—Body tissue usually located at the ends of long bones. Has a smooth, thick surface that provides some cushion and gliding surface for joints.

Center of gravity—The center about which a body would rotate if suspended. The center of the body.

Cerebrospinal fluid—Watery fluid that bathes brain and spinal cord; contained by the meninges.

Cervical—Referring to the neck.

Chin in—Exercise to improve neck posture done by pulling the chin backward.

Chin wipe—Exercise done to improve neck flexibility done by rotating the chin across the chest from shoulder to shoulder.

Chiropractic—Treatment discipline based largely on the theory that many symptoms and disorders may be explained by spinal malalignment. Basically, a different discipline from medical or osteopathic practice.

Chondral plate—Bone along the top and bottom surfaces of the body of each vertebra. Also called "end plate."

Chromotherapy—Relaxation techniques involving the use of imagined colors.

Circumduction—Circular rotating motion of a joint, usually applied to shoulder motion.

Cluster headache—Specific type of headaches that occur with rapid recurrences and long symptom-free periods.

Collagen—A protein formed in the body. Major component of scars, ligaments, tendons, and noncrystal portion of the bone.

Concavity—The inside or short side of a curve.

Conditioned—Ready because of experience and preparation.

Connective tissues—Tissues present throughout the body that act to bind one body part to another and fill the spaces between body parts.

Contrast material—Chemical used to fill spaces so they will show clearly on x-rays. Sometimes called "dye."

Contrast-relaxation exercise—Exercise to provide relaxation by first experiencing tension and then relaxation of certain muscles.

Cortex—Outer shell of bone. The hard, compact portion of a bone.

Cortisone—A chemical formed naturally by the adrenal gland. Among its many effects is a tendency to decrease inflammation. Many chemically similar drugs may be called cortisone, corticosteroids, or steroids.

Crick—Sudden catch in the neck that produces inability or reluctance to rotate or tilt the head in certain directions.

Curvature—A curve, bend, or portion of a circle. Variation from straight. Sometimes loosely used to mean the same as "scoliosis."

Degeneration—Changes that occur as a result of aging. May be a normal process or may be abnormal if it occurs faster or sooner than the normal aging process.

Deltoid—Muscle over the lateral aspect of the shoulder.

Diagonals—Lines joining opposite corners. In body mechanics, refers to lifting, pushing, and pulling forces where feet and arms are positioned so that the forces are taken diagonally through the body from one arm to the opposite leg.

Disc—Intervertebral disc. The joints between the vertebral bodies. Composed of a ring of ligaments (annulus fibrosus) and a center of semi-solid gel (nucleus pulposus). Sometimes spelled "disk."

Disc degeneration—Changes in the invertebral disc resulting in loss of volume and water content of the nucleus pulposus. Often accompanied by narrowing of the space that the disc occupies between vertebral bodies.

Disc space—Space occupied by the intervertebral disc. Located between the end plate of one vertebral body and that of the one adjacent to it.

Discectomy—Operation to remove a portion of an intervertebral disc.

Displacement activity—An action performed as a substitute for one that is feared or forbidden. For example, clenching the teeth instead of screaming out in anger.

Drop attacks—Sudden fainting spells, sometimes related to sudden changes in the circulation to the brain.

Dorsal—Portion of the back where the ribs are located. Between lumbar and cervical. Also called "thoracic." "Dorsal" can also be used to designate direction, in which case its meaning is nearly the same as posterior.

Dye—Term used to refer to certain contrast materials used in x-ray; for example, that used for myelograms.

Dysfunction—Absence of a normal function. Abnormal or irregular action.

Elasticity—Property of being able to increase in length under stress and then return to the original length at rest.

End plate—The bone along the top and bottom surfaces of the body of each vertebra. Also called "chondral plate."

Enthesis—The location of insertion of ligaments or tendons into bone. The interface between bone and the fibers that insert into bone.

Ergonomics—Study of body movement to perform work.

Estrangement—Alienation. Feelings of separation. Loss of trust and feelings of belonging with another person or group.

Extended—Brought out to form a straight line. Opposite of flexed. See "extension."

Extension—Extended, stretched out, straight position. Opposite of flexion. Sometimes may refer to motion beyond straight if opposite in direction to the direction of greatest action. For example, back bending as to look at the ceiling, while standing, is bringing the low back into extension.

Extracranial—Outside the skull.

Facet—Bony process on each side of the back of each vertebra.

Facet joint—Sites where the vertebrae join together at the back of the spine. Formed by one process from the vertebra above and one from that below on each side.

Fibromyositis—A term sometimes used to describe a syndrome which among other symptoms includes muscular fatigue, soreness, and tender areas.

Fribrosis—Condition of having an increase in the number of fibers and fiber cells in a tissue. Scarred.

Fibrous—Composed of fibers. Rope-like. In the body, usually containing a large amount of the protein collagen.

Flexed—Bent. Opposite of extended. See "flexion."

Flexibility—Ability to move. Freedom of movement as in joints of the body.

Flexion—Bent. Motion toward a bent position. Opposite of extension.

Foramen (pl. foramina)—Hole or window. Usually through or between bones.

Foraminotomy—An operation to enlarge the foramen.

Foraminal stenosis—Narrowing of the holes between the sides of the vertebrae (intervertebral foramina) so that the nerves that normally pass through these holes do not have adequate space.

Frontalis (frontal) muscle—Muscle across the front of the head controlling forehead expressions.

Fusion—An operation done to eliminate motion where it was previously present usually by removing bone from one area and placing it in the area to be fused.

Genitourinary organ—Organs of sex and of urine excretion. Kidneys, ureters, bladder, and uretha. Ovaries, uterus, and vagina in the female. Prostate, testicles, and penis in the male.

Gynecologic—Referring to the female reproductive organs.

Habituated—Having a strong desire for something though not an absolute physical need for it. For example, cigarettes among cigarette smokers.

Hamstrings—Muscles of the back of the thigh that cross behind the knee and hip.

Humerus—Bone of the upper arm.

Hypnosis—Technique of teaching discipline or relaxation by focusing the mind's attention upon the problem and placing of trust in the person providing the suggestions.

Hypoglycemia—Condition caused by drop in the level of blood sugar.

Ice massage—Application of ice over an area of soreness or muscle tightness along with pressure from the ice or from finger massage.

Inflammation—Reaction of the body or a part of the body to some kind of irritation. Characterized by swelling, increased temperature in the area, redness, and tenderness.

Intervertebral disc—The joints formed in the front of the spine where each vertebral body sits on the one below. Discs, composed of fibers and a gel, both cushion and support the vertebrae.

Intervertebral foramen—Hole between sides of each vertebra through which spinal nerves pass.

Intra-abdominal pressure—The pressure inside the cavity of the abdomen.

Intrathoracic pressure—The pressure inside the cavity of the chest.

Isometric—Without movement. Usually referring to exercises done by creating tension against resistance, without movement.

Joints—Areas in the body where bones join together. Motion may be almost none to a very wide range, depending on the location and characteristic of the joint.

Kyphosis—Curve of the spine in the chest area. The convex side of the curve is toward the back (posterior). Up to about 45 degrees of curve is normal.

Lamina—Portion of the vertebra that makes up the back roof over the vertebral canal. Each vertebra contains a right and left lamina from the spinous process in the middle of the facets and pedicle at each side.

Laminectomy—An operation to remove the back roof or "lamina" portion of a vertebra. Technically "laminectomy" means removal of the entire lamina structure of a vertebra, but the term most often is used to refer to any operation on the spine that approaches the contents of the vertebral canal from the back (posterior) side.

Lateral—To the side or from the side.

Lateral interbody joints—Areas of contact along the sides of the bodies of the cervical vertebrae, also called "uncovertebral joints" or "joints of vonLuschka."

Lateral tilt—Direct sideward bending of the head as though to put the ear on the shoulder.

Latissimus dorsi—Large muscle from the mid- and lower back inserting on the upper arm.

Ligament—Supporting structure from one bone to another. Formed of fibers.

Ligamentum flavum—Ligament that connects one lamina to the next, thus forming part of the "roof" of the back of the spine. Has a yellow color and unusual amount of elasticity. Also called "yellow ligament."

Lordosis—Forward curve of the lumbar (low back) area. The convex side of the curve is in the front (anterior). Also sometimes refers to forward curve present in the neck area.

Lumbar—Region of the back between the lowest ribs and the top of the pelvis.

Manipulation—A bending, twisting, or stretching action to attempt a favorable change in the position or movement of muscles, joints, or bones.

Mantra—Personal word or phrase used to produce relaxation or recall some other emotional attitude.

Mechanical back pain—Back pain occurring because the supporting structures of the back are not able to withstand the forces applied to them.

Median nerve—Large nerve passing along the palm side of the wrist into the hand, supplying the thumb side of the hand.

Meditation—Relaxation through attention to breathing or other solitary diversion from concerns over the stresses of life.

Meningeal sac—The container formed by the meninges. Holds the spinal fluid, spinal cord, and brain.

Meninges—Thin tissue coverings that encase the spinal cord and brain and the fluid that bathes them.

Menopause—Time of hormone changes of middle life.

Migraine headache—Specific form of headache, fairly common though less so than tension headaches.

Monosodium glutamate—Preservative used in Oriental and other foods that may produce headaches.

Motor points—Areas where nerves join muscles. May coincide with trigger points and acupressure points.

Muscle relaxants—Group of drugs used to relieve pain that is associated with muscle tension.

Myelogram—X-ray study in which a contrast material or "dye" is injected into the spinal fluid.

Nerve conduction test—Electrical test to determine the speed that an electrical impulse travels along a nerve.

Neurologist—Medical doctor who specializes in diagnosis and medical treatment of disorders involving the brain, spinal cord, and nerves.

Neurosurgeon—Medical doctor who specializes in diagnosis and care, including surgical operations, of disorders of the brain, spinal cord, and nerves. Also sometimes called "neurological surgeon."

Nerve roots—Nerves that join the spinal cord and course through the vertebral canal. Anterior and posterior roots at each level join to form a "spinal nerve."

Nitrites—Preservatives used in hotdogs and other meats which can occasionally cause headaches.

Nucleus pulposus—Central portion of the intervertebral disc. A semi-solid gel surrounded and contained by the annulus fibrosus and the bones of the vertebral bodies above and below.

Obesity—More than the desirable amount of body fat.

Obliterate—Eliminate. Dispose of. Remove.

Obliterate the lordosis—Flatten the lower back. Take the sag out of the low back. Pull in the abdomen. Do a pelvic tilt.

Occiput—Back of the head. Back and lower portion of the skull.

Orthopedic—Anything related to the correction of deformity and disorders of the spine, arms, and legs.

Orthopedic surgeon—Medical doctor who specializes in diagnosis and care, including surgical operations, of deformities and disorders of the arms, legs, and spine.

Osteopathy—Medical discipline originally based on spinal manipulation as a treatment for many disorders. Has evolved to be similar in principle to practice of medicine as practiced by medical doctors except the practitioners have a D.O. (doctor of osteopathy) rather than an M.D. (doctor of medicine) degree.

Osteophyte—Enlargement of a bone at its edge where ligaments attach to it. Sometimes called a "bone spur."

Overhead extension—Combination of shoulder motions used in reaching directly overhead.

Passive exercise—Exercise done wholly by the use of outside force without using your own muscles to participate in the exercise.

Pectoral muscles—Muscles of the front of the chest wall that attach to the upper arm.

Pedicle—Side wall portion of vertebra. Each vertebra has a right and left pedicle joining the body to the laminae and facets.

Pelvic bones—Bones that join to form the pelvis. The pelvis connects the thigh bones at the hip with the spine at the sacrum. The pelvis is formed from three bones grown together on each side—the ilium, ischium, and pubis.

Pelvic tilt—Rolling the pelvis forward and upward by flattening the lower back, pulling in and tightening the abdomen, and squeezing the buttocks together.

Pelvis—Lowest portion of the trunk. The pelvic bone has attachments for the hips and spine.

Pendulum effect—Force gained by pendulum-like swinging as in a grandfather clock. Frequently used in gaining shoulder motion.

Periscapular—Around the shoulder blade or scapula.

Plexus—Area where nerves interconnect.

Positive feedback cycle—Reactions that depend upon one another in such a way that an increase in one will lead to reactions in the others that will ultimately lead to further increase in the first one. This may be either for the good or for the bad. When for the bad, it is sometimes called a "vicious circle" or "vicious cycle."

Posterior—Toward the back. As opposed to "anterior" which means toward the front.

Prescription—Recommendation by a physician or other medical professional. Usually for medicine, exercise, or some other therapeutic effort.

Processes—When referring to bone, indicates outgrowths on the bone that serve as attachments for tendons and ligaments.

Prone—Lying face down, back up, on the abdomen.

Prostate—Gland in the male located between the back of the base of the penis and the rectum.

Protract—Elongate by arching forward. Used to designate the motion of the shoulder blade as the shoulder is thrust forward.

Psychotherapy—Treatment based on discovery of behavior and thought patterns and the causes of them. Usually practiced by psychiatrists, psychologists, or ministers.

Quadriceps—Muscles of the front of the thigh. Cross the front of the knee and hip.

Referred pain—Pain that is felt at a site distant from the source of its stimulus.

Rest position—Body position to relieve stress on a specific region of the body such as the neck or lower back.

Restorative—Restful. Bringing back to a state of feeling rested and having energy restored.

Retract—Pull back. Refers to the motion of the scapula that occurs across the chest as the shoulders are pulled back.

Rhomboids—Muscles from the back to the shoulder blades that provide retraction of the scapula.

Rheumatologist—Medical doctor who specializes in the diagnosis and treatment of arthritis.

Rotator cuff—Cuff of combined tendons from the shoulder blade to the upper arm that control shoulder motion.

Rotator cuff tendinitis—Inflammation in the tendons of the rotator cuff.

Rupture—A breaking out from the normal confines.

Scalenes—Small muscles that attach closely to the cervical spine.

Scapula—Commonly called shoulder blade. Large bone that connects the chest to the arm.

Scapula squeeze—Exercise done by retracting both scapulae.

Scar tissue—Body tissue with more than the usual amount of fibers as a reaction to injury or inflammation.

Scoliosis—A side-to-side (lateral) curve of the spine. If in a permanent, fixed position, it is an abnormal deformity of the spine.

Segment—A portion or section of anything. In the spine, it refers to two adjoining vertebrae with their enclosed disc and facet joints.

Shoulder blade—Large bone connecting the chest to the arm. The anatomic term is "scapula."

Shrugging—Pulling the shoulders up as though to touch the ears with the shoulders.

Spasm—Muscle tightness that is not under voluntary control.

Spinal cord—Extension of the brain from the base of the skull to the upper portion of the lumbar spine. Connects all the spinal nerves to the brain. Is located inside the meningeal sac, within the vertebral canal.

Spinal nerve—Nerve formed by the nerve roots from the spinal cord. Leaves the foramen and then either joins a plexus or continues as a peripheral nerve, depending on the location.

Spine—The bony structure of the back including the ligaments that bind together the 33 bones of which it is composed.

Spinous process—Posterior-most bone projection of the spine. Portion of the spine that can be felt through the skin.

Spondylitis—Inflammation of the spine. May refer either to infection or inflammation from other causes such as arthritis.

Spondylosis—Condition of the spine characterized by osteophytes, bone thickening, and disc degeneration.

Spondylotic myelopathy—Impairment of spinal cord function because of narrowing of the vertebral canal as a result of spondylosis.

Glossary

Spur—Rough edge on bone, or ligament that has turned to bone at the site of its attachment to bone. Also called "osteophyte."

Standing pelvic tilt—Flattening of the lower back, pulling in of the abdomen, and rolling forward and upward with the pelvis, while standing.

Stenosis—Narrowing of a hollow tube. When referring to the spine usually means narrowing of the vertebral canal or the intervertebral foramen.

Sternum—Bond in the middle of the front of the chest, commonly called "breastbone."

Sternocleidomastoid—Tubular muscles along the front of the neck from the sternum and collar bone to the skull.

Steroid—A group of chemicals, including cortisone, which have chemical structures and physiologic effects similar to hormones produced by the adrenal cortex.

Steroidal—Having the structure and properties of steroids.

Supine—Face up. Lying on the back.

Supine pelvic tilt—Flattening of the lower back, pulling in and tightening of the abdomen, squeezing the buttock muscles together, and tilting the pelvis forward while lying on the back.

Supine rest position—Reclining position on the back with the neck supported to relieve neck tension.

T.M.J.—Common abbreviation for temporomandibular joint.

T.M.J. syndrome—A combination of symptoms involving jaw muscle tightness and pain.

Target pulse—Pulse rate to produce improvement in general fitness without exceeding the range of safety.

Temporal artery—Artery on the side of the head above the ear.

Temporal muscle—Muscle along the side of the head.

Temporomandibular joint—Joint where the jaw joins the skull near the ear.

Tendon—Structure that attaches muscle to bone, sometimes called a "leader."

Tendinitis—Inflammation in or around a tendon, or at its junction with muscle or bone.

Tension—Tightness. Lack of normal ability to relax.

Tension headache—Commonest form of headache. Headache accompanied by tightness of the muscles of the face, head, and neck.

Thoracic outlet syndrome—Symptoms caused by pressure on the nerves and vessels as they pass from the neck into the arm.

Torticollis—Tilting and rotation of the head from spasm or disorder of the muscles or bones of the neck and head.

Tolerance (to pain)—Ability to withstand pain without loss of function or excessive need for care or compromise.

Traction—A pulling, stretching force usually used in attempt to relax muscles, assist in maintaining a proper posture, and stretch tight muscles, ligaments, or joints.

Tranquilizer—One of a group of drugs meant to decrease anxiety and relieve tenseness and fear.

Translational shift—Direct forward, backward, or sideways positioning of the head relative to the trunk or the trunk relative to the pelvis.

Trapezius—Large muscle from the neck to the scapula.

Trigger spot—An area of tenderness in the muscle that produces pain when pressure is applied to it.

Trunk—Central part of the body. Body except for arms, legs, and head. Torso.

Uncovertebral joints—Areas of contact along the sides of the cervical vertebrae which have some, though not all, of the characteristics of joints. Also called "lateral interbody joints" and "joints of vonLuschka."

Vertebra (pl. vertebrae)—Single bone component of the spine. Most people have seven in the neck (cervical), 12 in the chest (thoracic), five in the low back above the pelvis (lumbar), one large one composed of five fused together (sacrum) at the pelvis, and four or five small tail ones (coccygeal).

Vertebral canal—Tunnel through the spine from the head to the tail bone. Through it pass spinal cord and spinal nerves.

VonLuschka joints—Uncovertebral joints.

Vicious cycle or vicious circle—Series of actions and reactions in which the first thing that goes wrong leads to another or other things going wrong which in turn lead back to the first thing going further wrong.

Wall slides—Exercise done to strengthen the legs and the muscles of good low back posture.

Wryneck—Tilting and rotation of the head. Torticollis.

Yellow ligament—Ligament that connects one lamina to the next thus forming part of the back roof of the spine. Has a yellow color and unusual amount of elasticity. Also called "ligamentum flavum."

INDEX

Abdomen, 72, 122, 124–125
Acupressure, 9–10, 159
Alcohol, 44, 53, 60, 63, 66–68
Anatomy, 139–154
Annulus fibrosus, 141, 144, 147, 150
Arm pain and numbness, 7, 109, 164
Arthritis, 36, 45, 109, 167
Attorneys, 54, 88–93

Back:
   exercises, 115–117, 122, 124–125
   pain, 8, 115
Balms, 4, 5, 7
Bending, 27, 33
Bicycling, 128–129
Body language, 16, 18
Body mechanics, 26–42
   dressing table, 28
   of sex, 80–81
   workbench, 29
Bone composition, 140
Braces, 13

Carpal tunnel syndrome, 165–166
Chairs, 36–39
Chest pain, 163
Chin tuck exercise, 97
Chin wipe exercise, 112–113
Chromotherapy, 105

Collar, 13, 23, 87
Contrast relaxation exercise, 101–103
Crick, 4, 6
Cycles:
   neck pain-headache-neck pain, 155
   pain-demands-isolation-pains, 55–56
   pain-reward-pain, 53–54

Depression, 44, 49, 50, 53, 63–65, 127
Deep relaxation, 105–107
Diagonal principal, 31, 34
Diary, 54–55, 75
Diet, see Nutrition
Discs, 44, 143–152
   anatomy, 140, 143–145
   degeneration, 145
   shear effect on, 148–149
   surgery for, 150–152
Dizziness, 109, 153, 166
Diving, 85
Dressing table, see Body Mechanics
Driving, 24, 40–41
Drop attacks, 166
Ergonomics, 26–42
Exercises, 94–138
   active vs. passive, 110
   flexibility, 5, 23, 108–117, 162–163
   general fitness, 86, 127–136
   monitoring, 133–136

Exercises *(cont.)*
    posture, 16, 19, 96–99
    relaxation, 4, 51, 100–107
    sports and games, *see* Recreation
    strengthening, 21, 31–32, 118–126
    and weight control, 75

Facets, *see* Vertebra and Joints
Fear, 51–52, 87
Fibromyositis, 167
First aid, 1–13
Foramen, 142, 146–148, 150
Fusion operation, 151

Get tall (exercise), 19, 97–99
Glasses, 23, 24, 36, 167

Hair care, 45
Headrests (automobile), 41
Heat, 5, 7, 110
Headache, 156–159
    cluster, 157
    migraine, 80, 156–159
    posture as cause, 15
    sex related, 79–80
    tension, 47, 156–159
    treatment, 10, 14, 159

Ice, 4–5
Imagery:
    chromotherapy, 105
    getting tall, 19–20, 97–99
    guided, 57–59
    third eye, 19–20, 99
Insurance, 88–93
Intervertebral discs, *see* Disc
Isometric exercises, 118–120, 159

Jaw, 160–161
    exercises, 117
    muscle tension, 158, 160–161
Jogging, 128, 132–136
Joints, 140
    facet, 140, 146, 148
    intervertebral discs, *see* Disc
    uncovertebral, 141, 147, 150

Laminectomy, 151
Lifting, 27, 30–33
    down from a height, 34–36
    guidelines, 33

heavy, 30
intermediate, 31
light, 32
on the job, 33
setting objects down, 32
Ligaments, 140–142, 144
Lordosis, 72
Lying down, 21–23

Manipulation, 6
Massage:
    ice, 3, 4–5
    manual, 6, 159
    self, 2, 8, 161
Mattress, 22–23
Medicines, 14, 60–69
    acetaminophen, 14, 65
    addiction, 53, 62–63, 66–68
    antidepressants, 44, 62, 64–65
    anti-inflammatory, 61–62
    aspirin, 14, 61
    cortisone, 61
    muscle relaxants, 62–63
    pain relievers, 65–66, 68–69
    sleeping, 43–44
    tranquilizers, 62–64
Meditation, 103–105
Middle age, 49–50, 52–53
Mirrors, 26–27, 40
Mobilization, 6–8, 113–114
Motion:
    of neck, 110–111
    of shoulder, 114–115
Motor points, 9–10
Myelogram, 150

Neck rest positions, 2–4
Nerve conduction test, 166
Night pain, 44
Nucleus pulposus, 141, 144–145, 147–152
Nutrition:
    diet, 72–78
    dieting hints, 76–77
    overweight, 71–75
    vitamins, 70–71

Occupation, *see* Work
Osteophytes, 146, 150, 167
Overhead work, 34

Pain:
    as escape mechanism, 50
    as anger expression, 50–51
    exercise effect on, 48, 69
    first aid for, 1–13
    games, 56
    medicine effect on, 48
    nature of, 47–49
    tension as cause, 51
Pelvic tilt exercise, 97
Pillows, 2, 3, 22
Posture, 10–25
    exercises for, 96–99
    lying, 21–23
    overweight effect, 72
    sitting, 24–25, 39
    standing, 23
Psychological factors, 47–59
    adolescent, 16
    of dieting, 74–75
    middle age, 49–50
    of pain, 47–48
    self care for, 54–59
    of sex, 81–82
Pushing and pulling, 34

Reaching, 34
Reading, 24, 38
Recreation, 85–87
    dangers, 85–86, 120, 135–136
    dancing, 128, 130–132
    golf, 86
    riding, 87
    swimming and diving, 85–86
    tennis and racquet sports, 86
Relaxation exercises, 4, 51, 100–107
Rhomboid muscles, 121, 143
Rotator cuff tendinitis, 154, 161–163
Running, *see* Jogging

Scalene muscles, 143
Scapula, 153
    pain, 8
    pinch exercise, 16, 96, 121, 126, 165
Seatbelts, 41
Segments (of spine), 142
Setting objects down, 32
Sex, 80–84
Shear stress, 148–149
Shoulder:
    anatomy, 153–154

    exercises, 114–116, 119–123, 126
Shoulder blades, *see* Scapula
Sitting, 24–25, 36–39, 104
Sleeping:
    getting up from, 44–45
    medicines, 43–44
    posture, 22
    restorative, 43–44
Smoking, 46
Spasm, 6, 97
Spondylosis, 36, 45, 109, 152, 168
Sports, *see* Recreation
Spurs, *see* Osteophytes
Standing, 23, 26–29
State of mind commandments, 57
Stenosis, 147, 152
Stiffness, 108–117, 143
Stooping, 33
Supports, 13, *see also* Collar
Surgery, 150–152, 165, 166
Swallowing trouble, 167
Swimming, 85–86, 125–126, 129–130
Sympathetic nerves, 152–153, 166–167

Telephone posture, 39
Temperomandibular joint (TMJ), *see* Jaw
Tension:
    as cause of pain, 51, 81, 100, 158, 160
    control, 51, 101–107
Tension headache, *see* Headache
Theatres, 36
Thoracic outlet syndromes, 164–165
Torticollis, 6
Towel roll, 2, 7, 13, 22
Traction, 10–13
    door, 10–13
    manual, 6, 10
Trapezius muscles, 10, 121, 142, 158
Trigger spots, 9
Typing, 38–39

Vertebra, 140–142
    body of, 141, 144
    chondral plate (end plate) of, 145
    facets of, 146
    laminae of, 146
    pedicles of, 146
    spinous processes of, 146
Vertebral canal, 142, 146–147

Walking (for exercise), *see* Jogging
Weight, *see* Nutrition
Whiplash, 90–91
Work, 26–42, 88–90
  psychological value, 52–53
  restrictions, 30, 92

scheduling, 41–42
sitting, 36–39
standing, 26–27
Workbench, *see* Body Mechanics
Writing posture, 24, 29, 38
Wry neck, 6